Ageless Yoga

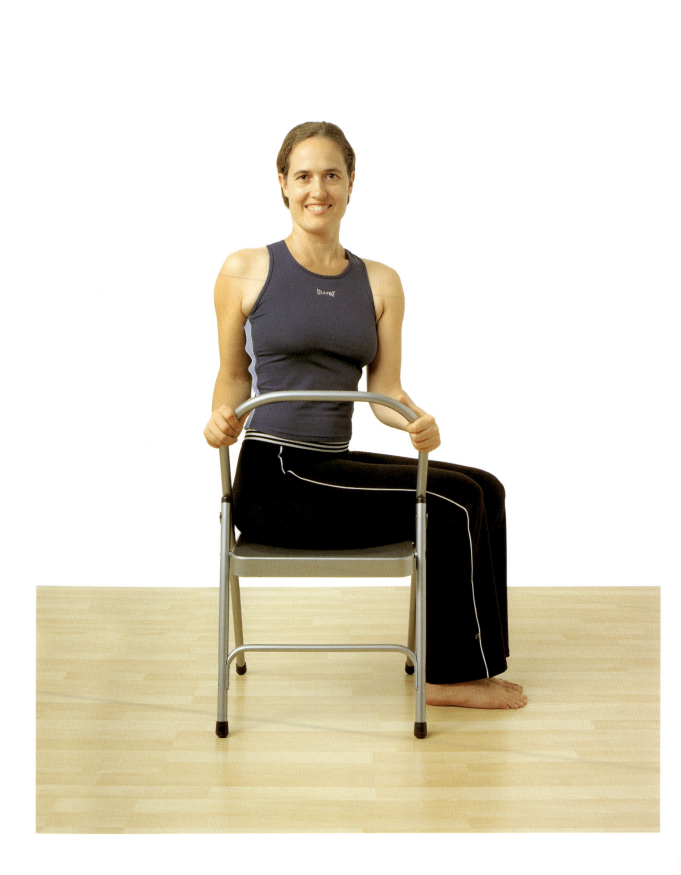

Ageless Yoga

Gentle Workouts
for Health & Fitness

JULIET PEGRUM

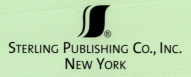

STERLING PUBLISHING CO., INC.
NEW YORK

AUTHOR'S ACKNOWLEDGMENTS

To all my kind teachers who tirelessly share their wisdom and to all who seek happiness
and freedom through the practices of yoga.

Juliet Pegrum can be contacted at: julietpegrum@mahamudrayoga.com

Library of Congress Cataloging-in-Publication Data Available

10 9 8 7 6 5 4 3 2 1

Published in 2006 by Sterling Publishing Co., Inc.
387 Park Avenue South, New York, NY 10016

Distributed in Canada by Sterling Publishing
c/o Canadian Manda Group, 165 Dufferin Street,
Toronto, Ontario, Canada M6K 3H6

First published in 2003 by Cico Books Ltd
32 Great Sutton Street London EC1V oNB
Copyright © Cico Books 2005

The right of Juliet Pegrum to be identified as author of this text has been asserted
by her in accordance with the Copyright, Designs and Patents Act of 1988.

Project editor: Mary Lambert
Photography: Geoff Dann

Printed and bound in Singapore
All rights reserved
Sterling ISBN-13: 978-1-4027-2377-3
ISBN-10: 1-4027-2377-6

IMPORTANT HEALTH NOTE

Please be aware that the information contained in this book and the opinions of the author are not
a substitute for medical attention from a qualified health professional. If you are suffering from any
medical complaint, or are worried about any aspect of your health, ask your doctor's advice before
proceeding. The publishers can take no responsibility for any injury or illness resulting from the advice
given, or the poses demonstrated within this volume.

Contents

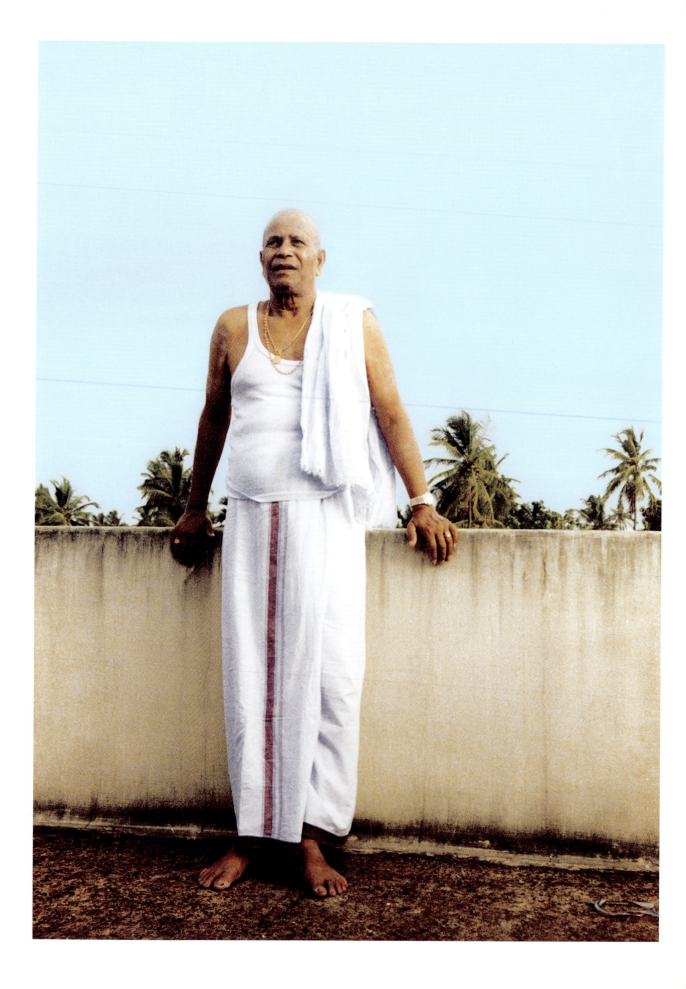

Age can make you either stupid or wise. Stupid means you
still hold on to lots of resentments; you wish you weren't getting old.
Yoga can lift that and bring wisdom and peace.

GURMUKH KAUR KHALSA

Introduction

Attaining eternal youthfulness and vitality has been the quest of scientists and philosophers the world over. Plastic surgery, high-impact exercise, and hormone replacement are just a few of the modern answers, sometimes with disastrous side effects. Yoga is a holistic approach that aims at prevention of illness, so that we can age naturally and with grace.

This book is designed to inspire those who wish to defy the conventional model of aging as a process of steady decline, and explore the potential for greater physical and spiritual awareness through the practices of yoga. According to yoga tradition, 50 years of age is the ideal time to develop physically and spiritually, because it is the stage in life when the children have grown, the mind naturally becomes more inward looking, and there is more time to dedicate to the study and practice of yoga. Man has a natural instinct to explore, and yoga is the perfect forum through which to explore the inner workings of the body.

YOGA AND LONGEVITY

Yogis living in India thousands of years ago unlocked the secrets of longevity. Yoga means to yoke or to join, to attach the mind to one object and to penetrate its essential nature. The object that the yogis chose was the human body. They studied intensely the internal activities of the body and mind like digestion, assimilation, expulsion, and breathing, so as to gain ever-greater understanding of its workings. In so doing they became masters of themselves; famous yogis like Krishnamacharya were able to stop their heartbeat at will. Many of the world's most renowned yogis like Indra Devi, B. K. S. Iyengar, Krishnamacharya, and Shree Pattabhi Jois continue practicing and teaching yoga into their 80s, 90s, and 100s, performing complex, mind-bending postures that we would consider impossible past a certain age.

Yoga is a lifestyle, not just a series of exercises. Gerontologists have recently confirmed that biological age can be speeded up or slowed down depending on lifestyle. They have found that adopting a healthy diet, regular exercise and a positive outlook on life can reverse ten years of the traditional signs of aging like high blood pressure, decreased muscle mass, brittle bones, and increased body fat. Slowing down the aging process begins with attention to lifestyle. By improving your diet and with a common-sense approach to maintaining fitness through yoga you can become stronger, increase flexibility, have more energy, and develop a positive outlook.

One of the paradigms of yoga is that "you are as old as your spine." Rounding or curvature of the spine is one of the first signs of aging, which is often accelerated by a sedentary lifestyle. Poor posture affects all the systems of the body, compressing the digestive organs, and restricting breathing. Yoga poses are designed to elongate and maintain the health of the spine and reverse bad postural habits. Also as we age, connective tissue begins to form across the long fibers that make up muscles, causing the muscles to shorten and harden, which affects the arteries. Stretching the muscles daily with yoga asanas breaks up the connective tissue, keeping the muscles soft, young, and supple.

YOGA AS MIND MEDICINE

As well as maintaining the physical body, yoga recognizes and cares for the energetic body (see page 10). According to the principles of yoga, health is experienced when there is an unimpeded flow of prana, or energy, within the body. Asanas combined with breathing and meditation exercises are designed to promote the free flow of energy throughout the body, resulting in greater vitality throughout life; with yoga, we can grow young.

How we think affects the flow of energy in the body. Yoga encourages us to become aware of the stream of life and to embrace and accept change, to focus our awareness on each moment as it arises and then to let it go. The body itself changes from moment to moment until after a seven-year cycle every cell in the body has been renewed. In yoga, it is believed that the more rigid we become in mind, the more rigid in body. Young minds are open and malleable, which is reflected in their natural physical flexibility. The life that flows within the body is like a mountain stream, constantly flowing. The life force is said to have always existed and to be indestructible. The yogi attaches his awareness to the life force, rather than identifying himself with the body and mind that are subjected to old age, sickness, and decay. Yoga helps us face all stages of life calmly yet courageously and encourages us to begin where we are now, in the present.

WHAT THIS BOOK CAN DO FOR YOU

Yoga is a timeless practice that brings body, mind, and spirit into ever-greater harmony. This book is a guide to the physical practices of yoga, including the poses, breathing exercises, and meditation for acquiring radiant health and tranquility. The beauty of yoga is that it can be practiced by anyone, regardless of age or physical ability. Many older students report that they feel in better shape after a few years of practicing yoga than they did in their 40s.

The principal chapters contain simple exercises for warming and limbering all the joints in the body, along with a range of props and exercise variations to make the poses more accessible so that the benefits can be experienced without strain. Asanas for Ailments

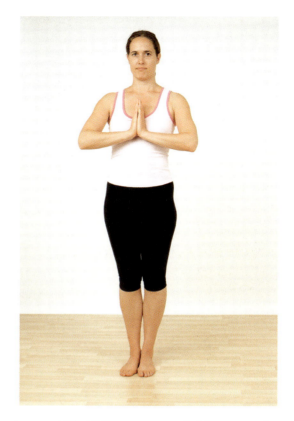

(pages 108–124), presents suitable poses for specific conditions, from improving flexibility in the feet to asanas that help with heart conditions, arthritis, and the menopause. A general workout is included as a guide for daily practice—20 minutes each day will bring you a sense of spontaneity, enjoyment, and well-being.

Yoga is not about self-improvement. It is about self-acceptance.

GURMUKH KAUR KHALSA

Diet

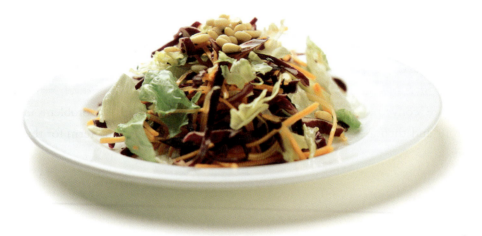

Yoga is more than a set of exercises: it is a complete lifestyle that includes proper eating habits. It is written in the Charaka Samhita that "the life span, complexion, vitality, good health, enthusiasm, plumpness, glow, vital essence, luster, heat and electricity (prana) are derived from the thermogenetic processes in the body," the main one being the "gastric fire." The gastric fire is considered the king of all the metabolic agents in the body, and it is said that proper maintenance of gastric fire is the basis of long life and vitality. There are two important factors in preserving this gastric fire: what we eat, and how we eat.

WHAT WE EAT

Nutrition is now recognized as one of the most important ingredients for prolonged good health. A poor diet high in sugar, animal fat, and sodium, and low in fiber can have disastrous health consequences, and doctors now attribute poor diet as a major contributor to many chronic diseases including heart disease, cancer, and diabetes. Obesity also impacts on the overall health of the body—as many as 40 percent of adults in the US are overweight.

THE YOGI DIET

Yoga's approach to diet is based on common sense. The yogis of old recognized that food contains a vital essence called *prana,* similar to the nutrients in food, which is essential to preserve life. Foods that have the highest level of prana are those that are closest to their natural state and source, for instance, an apple picked straight from a tree. An apple that has been packaged and then has sat around in the supermarket for a while has less vitality, and if it is then taken home and cooked, it loses a little more. In processed food, 90 percent of the nutrients are lost in the processing. That is why we often feel hungry soon after eating a large meal of processed food. The preferred diet of a yogi is one that is rich in natural unmodified foods such as fruit, vegetables, whole grains, nuts, and a little dairy produce. Sprouted grains are particularly high in nutrients as the starch and proteins are converted into nutrients to feed the sprout and then are passed easily into the bloodstream after eating.

Yogis tend to avoid eating meat because they believe in preserving life, and because meat is seen as having little nutritional value (the animal absorbs nutrients from grass and so eating the animal is considered a secondary, rather than primary, source of prana). Yogis also prefer foods that are light and are easily digested, whereas meat takes a long time for the body to break down and process.

However, in yoga it is also recognized that each individual has a unique constitution and requires a different combination of foods for optimum health. Food that is suitable for your body type should leave you feeling light and energetic and bowel movements should be regular and effortless.

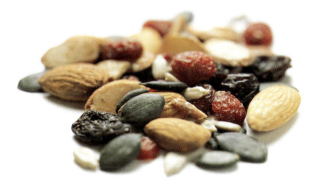

GOOD DIGESTION

Good digestion is recognized by the yoga system as a vital component to staying young and healthy. There is a saying in India that mental clarity comes from a straight spine and a clean colon. Many alternative health professionals also say that most chronic illness begins in the colon. Constipation and other bowel-related illnesses, like irritable bowel syndrome, are among the most prevalent problems in later life. In Indian philosophy, the term for the accumulation of toxins, undigested food, and waste material in the body is *Amma,* which is described as a sticky mucus that blocks the channels of circulation, causes irritable bowel, heaviness, lethargy, bad breath, and painful joints. *Amma* is viewed as a poison that slowly infiltrates the body causing it to break down. Chemically laden food and junk food are difficult for the body to assimilate, so they literally weigh down the body and poison the system.

To keep the digestive system streamlined, yoga advises eating only wholesome foods in smaller portions. When we overload the body with a heavy meal, it requires a lot of vital energy to process and assimilate the food. This takes energy away from being able to think clearly or be physically active, which is why we often feel dull and sleepy after a heavy meal. It is better to eat something light every 2 to 3 hours rather than three heavy meals. Plus as we age, the metabolism slows down and we require less food, although our eating habits do not change. If the system is particularly slow and sluggish, then fasting and internal colon cleansing are both recommended.

WATER

Drink lots of water between meals as this helps to hydrate the system, flushes the kidneys, assists cell function, reduces wrinkles, and helps with elimination of toxins.

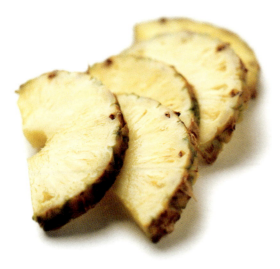

HOW TO EAT

Eating correctly includes how you eat and where you eat. It is important to be calm and relaxed while eating. In our fast-paced society, we are often forced to eat on the run or to grab a bite. Lunch breaks are getting shorter and we often find ourselves eating in front of the computer. When we eat quickly, we do not chew the food well, which is important as the majority of nutrients are absorbed in the mouth, so we are not getting maximum benefit from the food.

Eating a healthy diet does not have to be boring or tasteless. As you feel more energetic, eating the old way will no longer be appealing. Practicing yoga changes the body's cravings, and soon you will find yourself resisting junk food naturally.

Practicing the poses regularly aids the digestion. Many of the yoga asanas are specially designed to put gentle pressure on the colon and intestines, to remove excess gas, and to stimulate the digestive process.

GOOD POSTURE

Posture is important: sitting upright is not just a Victorian hang-up. When we slouch, the "gastric fire" is compressed and breathing, a vital component to digestion, is restricted, making it harder for the body to do the work of digestion and assimilation, causing a build-up of toxins. This is why it is good to take a short slow walk after eating, rather than slouching in front of the TV or going straight to sleep, as the upright posture assists the body's mechanism.

Yoga is not for him who eats too much, nor for one who absolutely abstains from food.
—Bhagavad-Gita VI -16

The Asanas

〜

Asana is the name for the postures of yoga. Yoga asanas include forward bends, backward bends, twists, balancing poses, and inversions. The postures help to tone the muscles and remove the built-up toxins in the body that can cause stiffness in the joints. The poses send oxygen and nutrient-rich blood to nourish every part of the body. The asanas aid digestion, increase circulation, improve concentration, boost the immune system, and generally increase strength and vitality.

FINDING HARMONY

It says in the yoga sutras that whether you are young, old or sick, if you can overcome inertia and laziness, success in the practices of yoga will be attained. Inertia is interpreted as the tendency of the mind to resist change. Humans are creatures of habit, and the older we become the harder it is to make changes and break negative habits. Simply starting yoga can be one of the most difficult obstacles to overcome, especially if you have not exercised in a long time, or are experiencing pain. Many people believe that they have to get fit before they can practice yoga, but the beauty of yoga is that it is available to everyone. The poses can be adapted to a person's needs with the use of numerous props. In yoga, change is embraced as we learn to move with the ebb and flow of life. The poses are difficult initially, because the body is working through a lifetime of habitual patterns of movement. The poses break down old patterns, and awaken new neuromuscular pathways in the brain; breakthrough is experienced as increased freedom and mobility. With regular practice, the poses will become steady and comfortable. Asana literally means steady, comfortable pose.

The body is designed to move in varied and complex ways. One only has to watch the beauty and grace of a ballerina to appreciate the body's potential range of movement. However, with modern life becoming increasingly compartmentalized, our range of motion is being constantly eroded. In the morning we get up from our comfortable mattress, then spend the day sitting at a desk, followed by an evening on a cushioned sofa. Many new injuries are surfacing due to the strain of limited repetitive movements, like carpal tunnel syndrome, which is caused by hours working on a computer.

Yoga practice not only conditions the physical body but it helps to develop our awareness. The presence and focus of mind required for the practice of yoga helps us to become more conscious of the actions that create stiffness in certain muscles and joints, and where we hold stress. Through yoga we can undo any negative postural patterns that contribute to pain and tightness, and return to natural alignment.

Alignment is not a matter of rigidly holding the body in line; rather it is a dynamic process that shifts with each movement. The key to good posture and alignment is that the muscles throughout the body are evenly toned. We tend to use the muscles more on one side of the body than the other, and the ones at the front more than the back. Yoga asanas exercise all the muscles in the body, even minor muscles, keeping the body in a state of dynamic alignment. That is why yoga stretches both sides of the body evenly, and builds muscle tone throughout the body. When the muscles are toned, the joints are fluid, the blood is circulating, the breath is even, and the mind is calm, the body returns to a state of harmony, free from pain.

HOW TO BREATHE

The ideal breath for asana practice is called *ujjai* breathing, whereby you gently contract the glottis to produce a soft snoring sound at the back of the throat while breathing. This action regulates the flow of breath, keeping it steady and even. Inhale slowly and deeply and exhale-completely, emptying the lungs without strain. The breathing should be soft, elongated, and rhythmic like the sound of the ocean. A simultaneous contraction of the abdomen should happen automatically, helping to protect the lower back.

YOGA AND SAFETY

A joint is the point where the end of two bones meet making articulation possible. Each joint is encased in synovial fluid and covered in cartilage, as lubrication is essential for joint mobility. Each joint has a natural range of motion. An inability to move a joint is due to an obstruction,

like a bone deformation, or the muscles that cross the joint being too tight. Stretching the muscles, and gently moving the joints to their full range of motion, as in the warm-up exercises, is the foundation of the yoga practice. Warm-ups prepare the body for the more complicated asanas.

Accidents most often occur due to the overzealousness of the student, who impatiently forces the body into a pose. Yoga has to be practiced with patience, intelligence, and awareness in order to avoid injury. In yoga there is no goal, there is only the journey. Moving in and out of the postures with awareness is just as important as the pose itself.

Always honor pain. A consistent stretching sensation means that the body is working and opening, but a sharp or uncomfortable pain is a signal from the body that something is wrong. If you do not listen to the body's warning signals, an injury may result. It is important to take responsibility for your well-being—even if a teacher tells you to do something but it feels

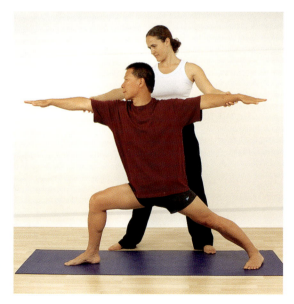

wrong, stop. Yoga is a system of self-knowledge: you have to be truthful and know your own capacity.

CARING FOR THE SPINE

Keeping the spine strong and supple is an essential part of yoga practice. With bad postural alignment the discs get compressed and can rupture or bulge, which is referred to as a slipped disc. The bulging disc can cause pressure on the nerves that results in severe pain, and block the communication between the brain and body, inhibiting movement. In adulthood, all the blood supplied to the spine is derived from movement, without which the discs shrink and lose their elasticity. All the yoga movements accentuate lengthening the spine and increasing the spaces between the discs. Back bends especially are useful for sending fresh blood to the discs and nerves located in the spine.

WHERE AND WHEN

If you are new to yoga or are recovering from illness, I strongly advise that you look for a qualified teacher to learn the basics. To progress, you need to have complete trust and faith in a teacher. It is worth taking your time to try different classes to find a teacher and style with which you feel comfortable.

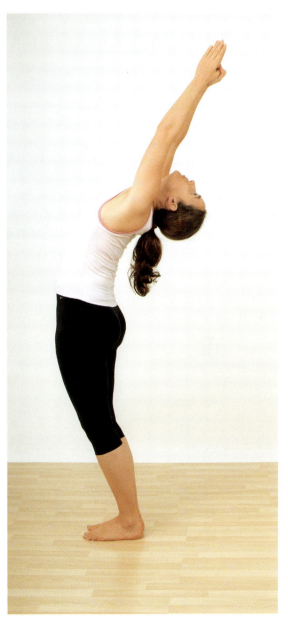

* Yoga can be practiced at any time of day as long as it is 3 hours after food and 1 hour after a caffeinated drink.
* Wear loose comfortable clothing.
* Practice in a warm, draft-free room, and if you are very stiff or suffering from arthritis then a hot bath or a heated room is recommended.
* The room should be clean, quiet, and free from distractions.
* Practice on a soft, slip-free surface. A yoga sticky mat is ideal.
* Anyone suffering from heart problems should not do any poses where the arms are raised over the head.

The mind is the maker and the mind is the destroyer.

—B. K. S. IYENGAR, *Tree of Yoga*

Thought Patterns

❧

Thoughts are like dynamite. The way we think directly impacts upon the body. In eastern medicine, it is said that all disease has a psychological component. Yoga has the basic principle of mind over matter, and sees the body primarily as a product of consciousness and secondly as a physical object, which is diametrically opposed to the western paradigm that sees the body as a biomechanical organism from which the mind springs.

THE MIND AND BELIEF

The body continually changes as a reflection of the mental state: How we think determines what we become. An image in the mind sends a powerful message through the entire nervous system. The nervous system is a complex network of information. Like a huge telephone exchange, it consists of the central nervous system, the brain and spinal cord, the somatic nervous system, which is in contact with the outside world, and autonomic nervous system that controls internal mechanisms like heart rate, or blood pressure. The thoughts running through the nervous system trigger hormones to be released into the blood which impact our physical body and appearance. When we are angry our face becomes red, the brow tenses up and the blood pressure rises. Recent scientific research has verified the link between the mind and the body; findings show that someone suffering from depression is four times more likely to develop disease. Depression or stress creates havoc with the immune system, sending a tidal wave of destructive hormones into the blood stream, which saps the life force. No thought or emotion is without electrochemical activity, which sends messages through which the body. The body is a field of energy in continual flux that is renewing itself every second.

Each time that someone asked Jesus to perform a miracle, Jesus would first ask the onlooker, "Do you believe?" Belief forms the bedrock in our minds of how and when things can happen. Believing yourself old, you will become old. In cultures that have a positive

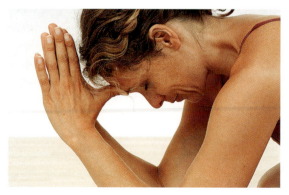

image of aging, a person is thought to become wiser with age and more able to lead the community, chronic age-related illnesses, like heart attacks and arthritis, are relatively nonexistent. Aging is fluid and changeable, which continually baffles scientists, as there is no consistent pattern. Each person experiences aging differently, depending on their response to the external world, which in turn influences their mental state.

Negative thoughts produce negative results. The way we think affects the body's nerves, glands, and energy channels. Negative thoughts choke and stifle the flow of energy through the channels; positive feelings like joy or love cause the energy channels to open, which is why we feel a rush of energy and are more buoyant and energetic when in love. Positive thinking and affirmations are an integral part of yoga practice, as a way to redirect mental energy and trigger a constructive chemical response in the body. Eric Shiffman, *Yoga: The Spirit of Practice and Moving Into Stillness*, says "When you catch yourself imagining an undesirable future like, 'my health will just get worse,' be aware you are thinking this, pause, cancel the thought, and take a moment to feel the creative life force which is what you are. Don't believe the negative projections; instead feel the energy that constitutes you. This way you leave a space for the miraculous to occur."

In my experience I find that many people who enter a yoga class have already decided what they can and cannot do before they even start a pose. But I cannot stress enough the importance of an open mind. When the mind is

According to yoga scripture, the body is made of five layers, like an onion, each level more subtle than the previous one:

1. Annamaya Kosha: the physical body

The physical body is considered to be the aspect of ourselves with which we most identify.

2. Pranamaya Kosha: the energy body

The energy body is made up of a network of 72,000 energy channels, or *nadis,* that span our entire bodies, the channels radiating from certain energy centers called *chakras,* meaning wheels. The energy that moves through the channels is called *prana,* or life force; it is like a wind that moves and animates the physical body.

3. Manomaya Kosha: the mind body

Our thought patterns determine how energy flows through the body. Thoughts are said to be like a subtle vibration that stirs the inner winds or energy body that then incites the body into action.

4. Vijnanamaya Kosha: awareness

Awareness is a field of pure perception, which can be experienced during deep meditation as a silent witness to our thoughts and reactions.

5. Anandamaya Kosha: the field of limitless potential The energy moves from the center outward just like the concentric ripples on the surface of a pond from the field of potential out to the physical body.

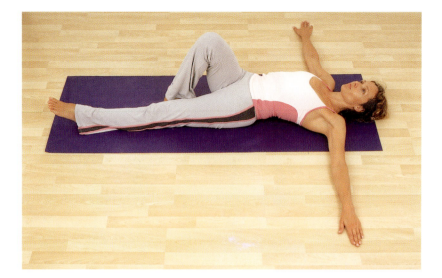

present in each moment free of expectation, then miracles can happen and the body can move in new and unfamiliar ways.

The purpose of yoga is to harness the tremendous energy of the mind. The poses and the breathing techniques deliberately open and redirect the flow of energy that in turn calms the mind and changes habitual ways of thinking. When the energies of the mind are harnessed through meditation they can be directed toward accomplishing any goal. The complicated movements of yoga are the first step in training the mind, through developing concentration. Concentration is necessary to carry out the complicated movements, and to hold the poses. Even thinking about performing an exercise has

benefits: when you think about a certain area of the body electrical impulses increase in that area. For someone in too much pain to do the physical asana, just visualizing the poses has a positive effect and promotes healing. The medical community, with startling results, has studied the effects of biofeedback. Using a biofeedback machine, doctors have shown that it is possible to control and change such autonomic body functions as blood pressure, heart rate, circulation, digestion, and perspiration. A positive, kind attitude toward your body is important. Even if it is causing you pain and you are frustrated, sending positive thoughts helps to change negative patterns and promote healing.

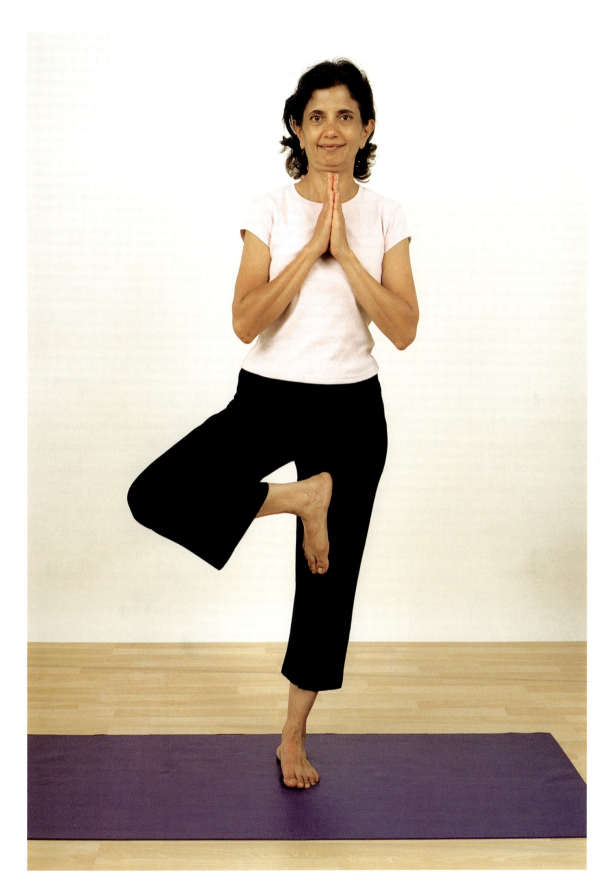

CALMING PRANAYAMA

Rhythmic Breathing

Rhythmic breathing reflects the way that babies breathe and the breathing pattern during deep, relaxed sleep. This breathing technique uses the diaphragm and minimizes the action of the rib cage. The technique activates the lower lobes of the lung while the action of the diaphragm also massages the liver and stomach and aids digestion.

This is a very simple, calming breath. It is a useful exercise while lying in bed to aid sleep.

Place one or both hands on the belly. As you inhale, gently relax the belly until you feel the belly pushing against your hands. On the exhalation, draw the belly back toward the spine. This breath can be practiced for as long as it is comfortable.

Full Yogic Breath *Deergha Swaasam*

Full yogic breath is an extension of rhythmic breathing, whereby the inhalation and exhalation is lengthened with the use of the rib cage. Indra Devi, the first lady of yoga, who lived and practiced yoga daily until aged 102, recommended 60 deep breaths a day. It takes time to build up the intercostal muscles and the lungs, so take it slowly and build up over time and start with a few rounds.

Breathing deeply comprises a three-step process.

1. Inhale by expanding the abdomen, drawing air to the lower lung.

2. Expand the rib cage out to the sides taking air into the middle of the lung.

3. Lift the collarbones, bringing air to the top of the lung. Exhale in reverse order, releasing the breath from the upper lung, middle lung, and then drawing in the belly. Make both the inhalation and exhalation one continuous flow. Repeat the breath 3 to 5 times, end on an exhalation, then return to normal breathing.

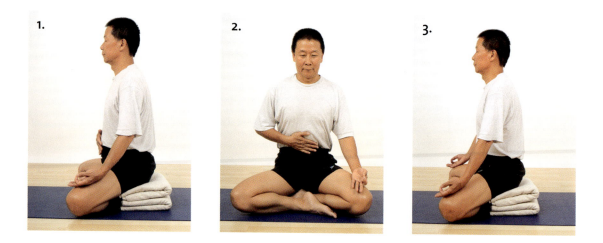

1.   **2.**   **3.**

Nerve Purification Breath *Nadi Suddhi*

In this technique, the breath is through alternate nostrils, which is a very powerful method of calming and relaxing the nervous system. When we breathe through the right nostril, which is called surya, *the sun channel, it activates the left side of the brain, which governs the sympathetic nervous system. When we breathe through the left nostril,* chandra, *the moon channel, the right side of the brain is activated. By breathing through alternate nostrils, the nervous system is brought into harmony and balance.*

1. Sit on the floor in a comfortable meditation posture with the spine erect. Bend the right arm and take the right hand into *Vishnu mudra* by closing the forefingers and index fingers. Relax the face.

Close the right nostril with the thumb. Completely exhale all the air from the lungs through the left nostril without strain, then slowly and deeply inhale through the same nostril to the count of four. Expand the stomach and chest to pull in more air, without strain.

2. Next close the left nostril with the ring finger and release the right nostril. Very slowly exhale making the exhalation longer than the inhalation. With practice, the exhalation should be twice the length of the inhalation, but do not rush it. Then inhale through the same nostril, close the right nostril and open the left nostril and repeat the cycle. Perform at least ten rounds. Release, and return to normal breathing.

Vishnu Mudra

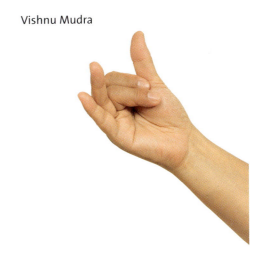

1.

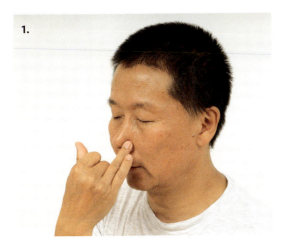

2.

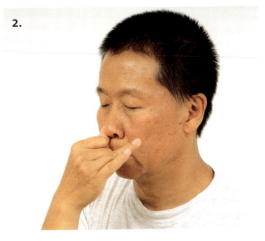

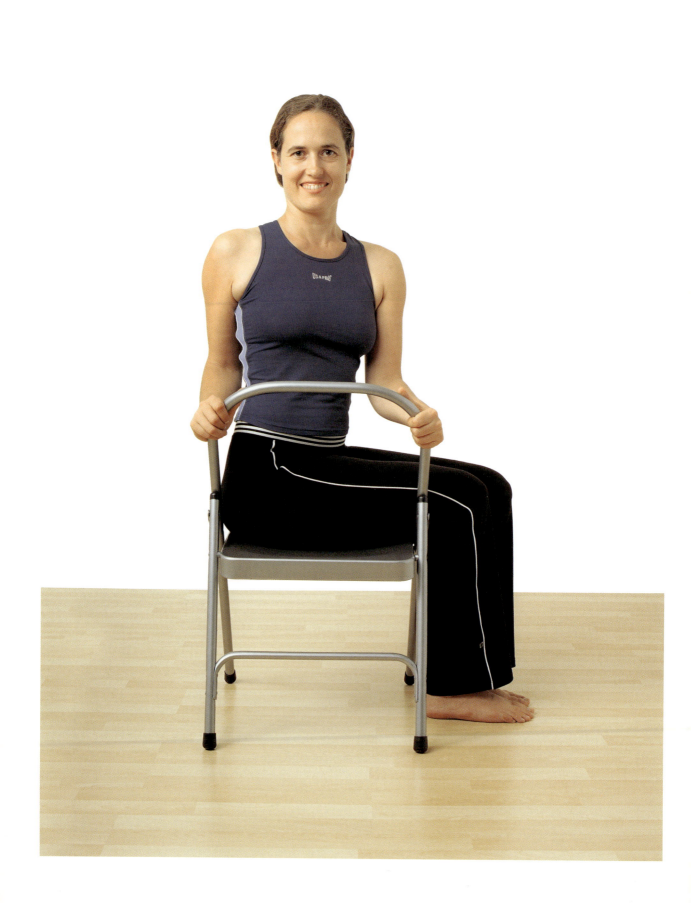

CHAPTER I

Working with Props

The use of props was pioneered by the great Indian yogi B. K. S. Iyengar, and has since been adopted by many schools of yoga. A prop can be any object as long as it is sturdy, will support the required weight, and helps you to practice a pose safely. Props are especially useful for beginners, or anyone with injuries, because they help you navigate around old injuries, allowing the body to experience a pose in an open, more relaxed way. Using a supportive prop also gives the nervous system time to become accustomed to a pose, so that later it may be practiced more easily. Many experienced yoga practitioners also enjoy using props as part of restorative practice, which involves using gentler versions of complete poses. Props allow you to hold the poses for much longer, without undue strain.

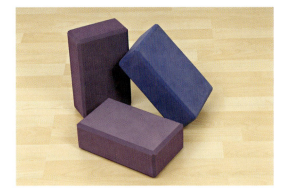

Blocks

Yoga blocks are made of wood or lightweight foam. Blocks can be used in myriad ways and are especially useful for people with less flexibility, allowing them to practice the poses without strain.

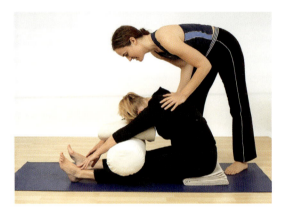

Bolster

A bolster is a long firm cushion that is a perfect prop for a range of restorative poses. Restorative poses are gentle, relaxing adaptations of complete poses that are useful when a person is low in energy, experiencing a life change such as menopause, or if recovering from illness or injury.

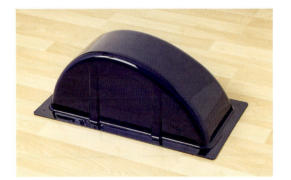

Back arch

A back arch is a great way to gently flex and elongate the spine without fear of injury. Lying over an arch provides the perfect counter-stretch after a day working at a desk. The back arch gently arcs over into a deeper curve.

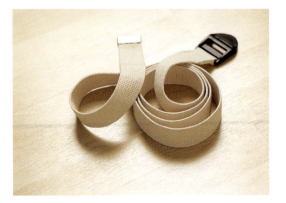

Belt

A belt is useful for new practitioners, helping users to extend their reach and easily access poses like forward bends, or other poses in which the hands need to reach the feet or clasp together behind the back.

Blanket

A blanket is a great basic prop—you can easily fold it to allow for additional lift and height in forward bends and shoulder stands, as well as using it as a cover to keep the body warm during relaxation.

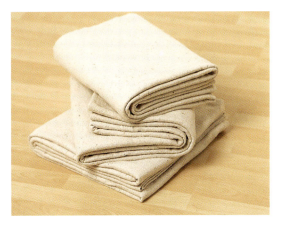

Chair

A chair is one of the most versatile props, especially for those who are stiff and new to yoga and have difficulty sitting on the floor, or getting down to or up from the floor. A chair helps maintain balance for older practitioners who fear falling; it also promotes the necessary strength so that you become less dependent upon it. A regular metal fold-up chair is best. Choose one that is robust with a large enough gap between the seat and the back rest to allow the legs to slide easily through the back.

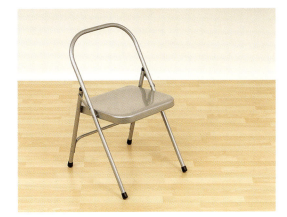

Wall

A section of bare wall is perhaps the simplest of props, and the perfect teacher of alignment. Standing in *tadasana,* with the back to the wall, helps us discover how far we have strayed from an upright position. A wall is a great support for inversions, providing a useful way to ease into shoulder stand, and a support for both handstand and headstand.

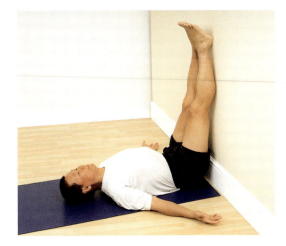

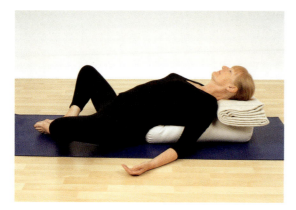

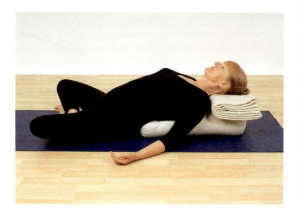

Cobbler pose with a bolster
Supta Baddha Konasana

Sit in *dandasana* (see page 79). Place a bolster behind you, lengthwise, and have ready a folded blanket by your mat. Bend the knees and draw the soles of your feet together, close to the groin. Relax the knees out to the sides; inhale. Exhale, lie back on the bolster so that the ribs are supported and the spine is on the center of the bolster. Place the blanket under the head to relieve neck tension. Tuck the chin in slightly, to extend the back of the neck, and relax the face. Relax the arms out to the sides, palms up, and the shoulders relaxed down. To deepen relaxation, inhale slowly and deeply and exhale slowly, emptying the lungs without strain. Breathing should be soft, elongated and rhythmic like the sound of the ocean. Hold for 5 to 10 minutes.

BENEFITS Using a bolster in *supta virasana* or *baddha konasana* can help during menopause as they release the pelvis and regulate hormone production; these poses also aid digestion.

✳ **TIP** If the legs are uncomfortable in *baddha konasana,* then simply cross the feet at the ankles to form *sukhasana.*

Hero pose with a bolster *Supta Virasana*

Kneel on the mat. Place a bolster on the mat behind you so that the top of the bolster touches the base of the ribs. Lift up onto the knees and separate the feet. Gently sit back and ease the buttocks down between the feet. If you experience strain in the knees, place a folded blanket under the buttocks or widen the knees. Gently lower down onto the bolster so that the spine is on the center of the bolster. Place a folded blanket under the head for additional support. Breathe deeply and rhythmically. Hold the pose for 5 to 10 minutes.

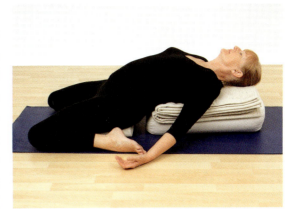

Downward dog with a bolster

Adho Mukha Svanasana

Place a bolster on the mat lengthwise. Come onto all fours with hands palms down on either side of the bolster, close to the far end. Tuck the toes under, inhale, and push up into downward dog. Relax the head and shoulders and place the forehead on the bolster. Breathe steadily; hold for 5 to 10 minutes. Exhale to come down.

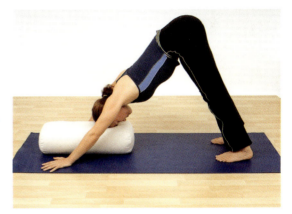

✳ **TIP** If you experience strain in the knees when lowering down onto the bolster, raise the height of the bolster using folded blankets.

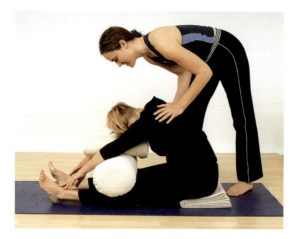

Forward bend with a bolster

Paschimottanasana

Sit in *dandasana* (see page 79). Place a bolster across the legs. Inhale, lift up and elongate the spine. Exhale and bend forward, placing the forehead on the top of the bolster. Relax the arms over the bolster to form a gentle forward bend. Breathe steadily and easily. Hold for 5 to 10 minutes.

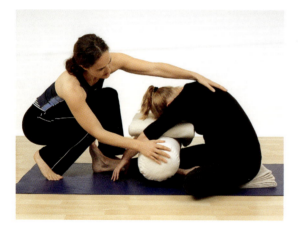

Head-to-knee pose with a bolster

Janu Sirsasana

Sit in *dandasana* (see page 79). Bend the left leg and place the sole of the left foot along the inside of the right thigh. Place a bolster across the extended left leg. Inhale, lift up and lengthen the spine. Exhale and bend forward over the extended leg. Place the forehead on top of the bolster. Relax the arms forward over the bolster. Breathe steadily and evenly. Hold for 5 to 10 minutes, then repeat on the opposite side.

BENEFITS Relaxing the head forward rests the heart and sends a supply of oxygen-rich blood to the brain.

✳ **TIP** If it is not possible to place the forehead easily on the bolster, place a folded blanket on top of the bolster for added height.

Side twist with a chair *Bharadvajasana*

Sit sideways on the chair, with the back of the chair in the direction of the twist. Place the ankles directly under the knees with the feet and knees together. Inhale, sit up, lift the chest and elongate the spine. Exhale and turn to the right. Hold the chair back with both hands, and use the back of the chair to pull deeper into the twist. Twist from the base of the spine, then the navel and the chest. Look over the right shoulder and hold for 8 breaths. Repeat on the opposite side.

BENEFITS Both the side twist and the forward bend with a chair are invaluable poses for anyone suffering from back stiffness.

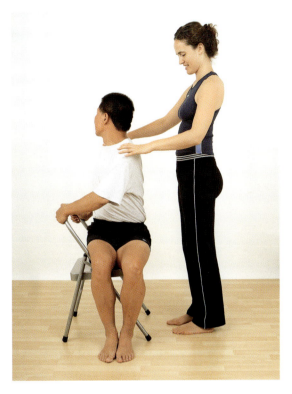

Forward bend with a chair *Uttanasana*

Sit on a chair so that the buttocks are close to the back of the chair seat. Place the feet on the outsides of the front chair legs, so that the soles of the feet are flat on the floor. Inhale and elongate the spine, then exhale and fold forward between the knees and relax the upper body down over the front of the chair. Relax the neck and shoulders. Now hold the pose for a few minutes, breathing evenly. Slowly curl up, one vertebra at a time.

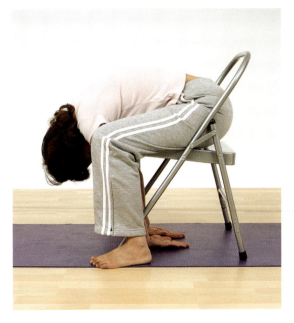

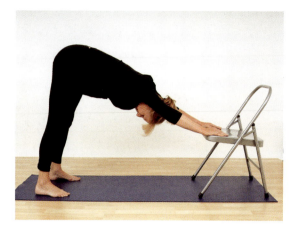

Downward dog with a chair

Adho Mukha Svanasana

Place a chair at one end of the yoga mat with the seat facing toward you. Inhale, then exhale as you bend forward, placing the heels of both hands so that they rest at the front edge of the chair. Walk the feet backward about 3 to 4 feet (1 to 1.2 m) from the chair. Now press away from the front of the chair with both hands, and lift the pelvis high. Flatten the back and look down between the arms. Hold the pose for 20 to 30 seconds, breathing evenly, then exhale as you release and come down.

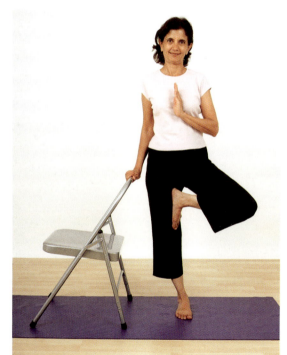

Tree pose with a chair *Vrksasana*

Place a chair on the mat and stand next to it with the back of the chair toward you. Come into tree pose using the back of the chair for support, slowly lifting and bending the left leg up and out to the side then resting the sole of the foot on the right thigh. Hold for 8 breaths then repeat on the opposite side.

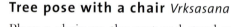

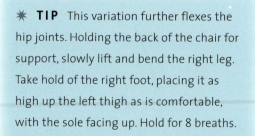

✳ **TIP** This variation further flexes the hip joints. Holding the back of the chair for support, slowly lift and bend the right leg. Take hold of the right foot, placing it as high up the left thigh as is comfortable, with the sole facing up. Hold for 8 breaths.

Plow pose with a chair *Halasana*

1. Place a folded blanket on the mat and chair seat; place the chair next to the blanket, so the front legs touch the edge of the blanket. Lie on the blanket with the shoulders parallel to its edge and the head underneath the chair seat. Place the hands alongside the hips, with the palms face down. Inhale, and on an exhalation bend the knees in toward the chest and swing the legs up over the head. Support the back with both hands.

2. Extend the feet through the back of the chair and place the tops of the thighs on the seat of the chair. Once the legs are supported release the hands and extend the arms on the floor away from the feet.

3. Interlock the hands and stretch the arms away to come higher onto the shoulders. Relax the face. Breathe steadily and hold for 1 to 3 minutes.

4. To release, slowly roll out, supporting the buttocks with the hands. Relax, with the knees toward the chest.

1.

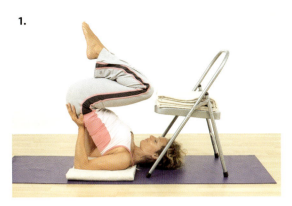

2.

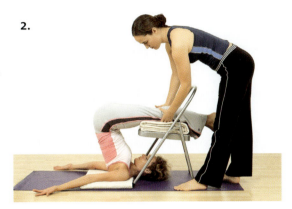

3.

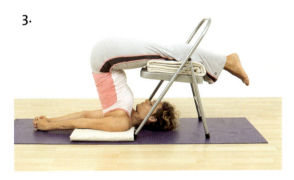

4.

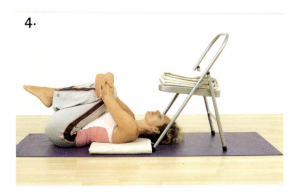

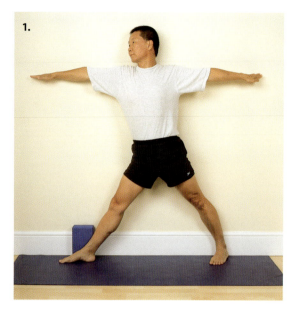

Triangle pose with a block *Trikonasana*

Blocks can act as useful hand rests in most standing poses. Place the block on or near the mat, within easy reach.

1. Stand in *tadasana* (see page 60). If you need to, rest the back against a wall for additional support. Step the feet 3 to 4 feet (1 to 1.2 m) apart. Rotate the right foot and leg out toward the end of the mat and turn the left foot into a 45-degree angle. Keep the pelvis facing forward. Place the block on the outside of the right ankle. Inhale, lift the arms to shoulder height, and extend out to the fingertips.

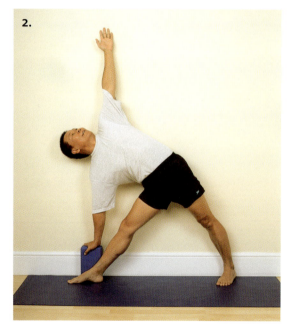

2. Exhale and lean to the right, keeping the chest and pelvis facing forward. Place the right hand on the top of the block. Extend the left arm up, so that the arms form a vertical line. Turn the head to look up toward the left hand. Hold for 8 breaths. Repeat on the opposite side.

BENEFITS Triangle poses remove stiffness in the legs and hips, stretching the intercostal muscles of the ribs, which helps to improve breathing capacity.

Bridge pose with a block

Setu Bandhasana

Bend the legs, stretch the arms toward the feet, and hold the ankles. Tuck the tailbone under; inhale. Exhale, pushing into the heels and lifting the pelvis. Roll onto the shouldertops and lift the chest. Place a horizontal block underneath the sacrum. With the arms relaxed, tuck the chin to gently stretch through the neck. Hold for 8 breaths. Exhale, lift the pelvis (see right), remove the block. Release, relaxing one vertebra at a time.

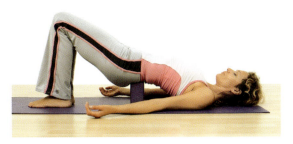

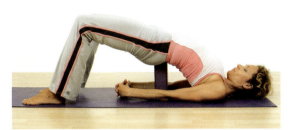

✹ **TIP** If you are comfortable with the block placed horizontally, and depending on the flexibility of your spine, you can place the block vertically. Clasp the hands and push down with the arms and sides of the hands to raise the pelvis higher, then ask a partner to position the block vertically.

Cobbler pose with blocks

Baddha Konasana

Sit in *dandasana* (see page 79) with the legs outstretched. Bend both knees and bring the feet in toward you as close to the groin as possible. Touch the soles of the feet together, and drop the knees to the sides. Place a block underneath each knee for support. Hold the feet and keep the spine straight and lifted. Hold the pose for 20 to 30 seconds or longer, breathing evenly.

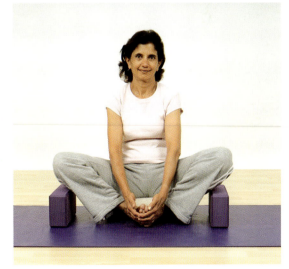

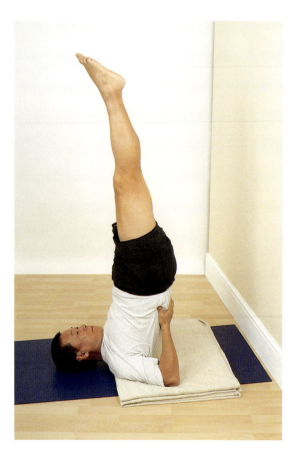

Shoulder stand with a blanket
Salamba Sarvangasana

Fold a blanket so that it is wide enough for the shoulders. Make sure that the edge of the blanket the shoulders are against is neatly folded and straight. Lie on the blanket so that the tops of the shoulders are in line with the edge of the folded blanket.

Tuck the chin in slightly and lengthen through the back of the neck. Place the arms alongside the body with the palms down. Exhale and bend the knees. Push into the palms and begin to raise the legs over the head. Bend the arms and place the hands in the middle of the back on either side of the spine to support the back, without widening the elbows.

Bring the torso to a vertical position moving the chest toward the chin. Straighten the legs to a vertical position, in line with the torso. Aim for a straight line between the shoulders, hips, and ankles. Tuck the tailbone under and lengthen along the spine. Remember to relax the muscles in the face. Stay breathing quietly for at least one minute. Come down carefully by placing the palms of the hands down flat on the floor and rolling down slowly, one vertebra at a time.

✳ TIP Most people are stiff in the lower back and hips, which means that when they sit directly on the mat, the base of the spine tends to bow outward.

To compensate for the tightness, sit up on a folded blanket so that the hips are higher than the knees, in order to protect the lower back during forward bends like *paschimottonasana* and *janu sirsasana* (see pages 81, 82).

Half-lotus *Ardha Padmaasana*

Sit on a folded blanket or block to raise the hips and ease the lower back. Bend the left leg and place the left foot close to the groin with the sole of the foot facing up. Bend the right leg and, carefully taking hold of the ankle, lift the right foot up over the left leg and onto the top of the left thigh with the sole of the right foot facing up. Lift the chest, lengthen the spine, and place the hands on top of the knees. Hold for 20 to 30 seconds. Release the legs and repeat on the opposite side.

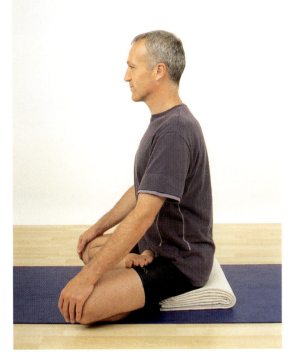

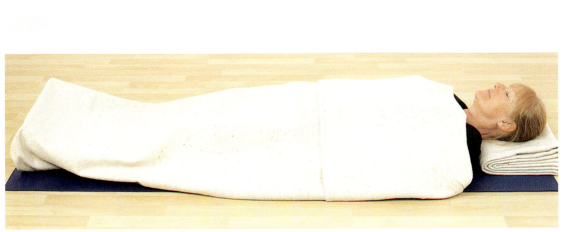

Savasana with a blanket *Savasana*

After practicing yoga asanas it is highly recommended that you rest for ten minutes in *savasana*. This pose, in which you lie comfortably on your back, gives the body time to deeply relax and absorb the full benefits of the practice. Also, because the body's temperature rises during the practice and the muscles become warm, it is important not to lose heat too quickly from the body as this causes shock to the system. Unless it is a really hot day, always wrap up for *savasana*—put on socks and a cardigan, if you have one with you, and cover yourself with a blanket—to retain heat, as the body temperature drops dramatically during relaxation.

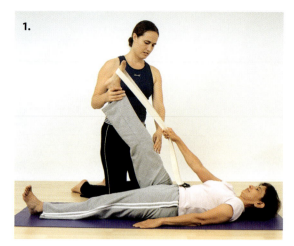

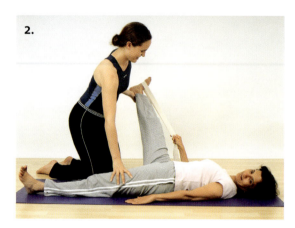

Lying thumb-to-foot pose with a belt

Supta Padangusthasana

1. Lie flat on the back with legs and feet together. Bend the right leg in toward the chest and place a belt around the ball of the right foot.

2. Take hold of both ends of the belt with the right hand. Straighten the right leg up, stretching into the heel of the right foot. Keep the right shoulder down, the hips level, and the left leg strong by pushing into the ground with the left thigh. Keep the left arm alongside the body with the palm down. Inhale. Exhale and extend the right leg out to the right side as far as is comfortable. Turn the head to look over the left shoulder. Hold for 8 breaths. Repeat on the opposite side.

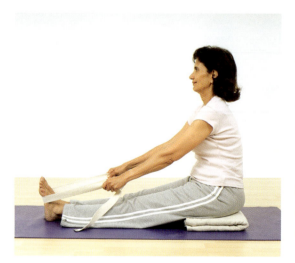

Seated forward with a belt

Paschimottanasana

Sit in *dandasana* (see page 79). Bend the knees and place a belt around the balls of both feet, then straighten the legs. Inhale; lift the chest and elongate the spine. Exhale. Bend forward with a flat back and grasp the belt as close to the feet as possible. Take the elbows to the sides and the head toward the knees. Relax the back of the neck and shoulders. Keep the thighs pressed into the floor. Hold for 8 breaths. Inhale and come up.

Tree pose with a belt *Vrksasana*

Stand in *tadasana* (see page 60) and spread the toes. Begin to take the body weight into the left leg. Bend the right leg and place a belt around the right ankle so that the belt wraps around the thigh. Use the belt to lift the foot as high as possible and place the sole of the foot on the inside of the left leg. Keep hold of the belt with the right hand. Hold for 8 breaths, breathing steadily and evenly. Repeat on the opposite side.

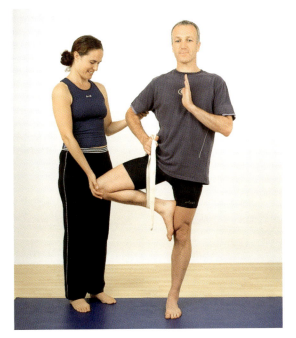

✳ **TIP** An alternative to wrapping the belt around the ankle and thigh is to loop one end of the belt. Slip the loop over the right foot and onto the right ankle. Gently use the other end of the belt to lift the right leg up and place the sole of the right foot as far as possible on the inside of the left leg.

Cow-face pose with a belt

Gomukhasana

Sit with the legs out straight. Bend the left leg so the knee is in line with the center of the body. Place the heel on the floor by the right hip. Bend the right leg over the left, so that the heel is in line with the left hip.

Holding a belt in the right hand, raise the right arm. Bend the right elbow and reach the right hand behind the back of the neck. Bend the left arm behind the back at waist level and grasp the belt. Work the left hand closer to the right hand using the belt. Keep the head and neck straight. Hold for 8 breaths, breathing evenly. Repeat on the opposite side.

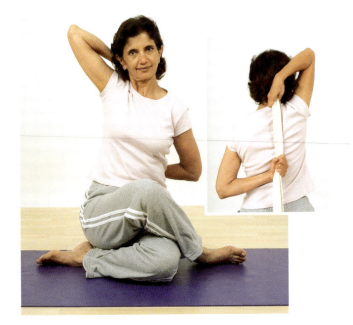

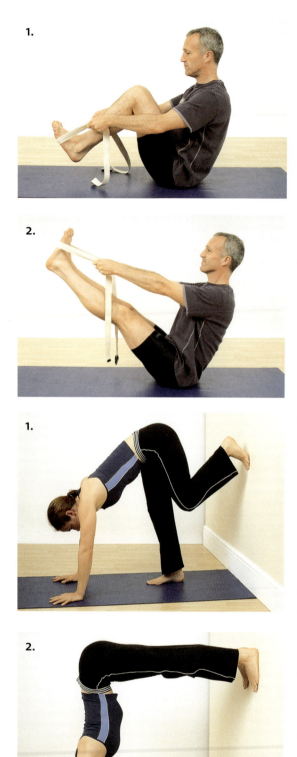

Boat pose *Navasana*

1. Sit with your legs outstretched in front. Bend the knees and place a belt around the balls of the feet. Hold the belt in both hands and slowly lean back until you are balancing on your buttocks.

2. When you are balanced, inhale then exhale as you slowly straighten the knees and extend the legs. Keep hold of the belt. Draw in the belly and lift the chest. Hold for 8 breaths, breathing evenly in the pose.

Half-handstand with a wall
Ardha Vrksasana

1. Practice the half-handstand using a wall for support as a way to build up the strength and confidence necessary for the full handstand. Stand with your back to the wall. Squat down and place the hands on the mat about 3 to 4 feet (1 to 1.2 m) from the wall. Raise the hips. Bend the left knee and place the sole of the left foot on the wall at hip height.

2. Shift the body weight into the hands. Press the left foot into the wall and lift the right foot up in line with the left foot. Press into both feet and straighten the legs to form a right angle between the legs and the torso. Hold for 10 to 20 seconds and carefully come down one foot at a time. Return to a squatting position for a few moments before standing.

Handstand with a wall

Adho Mukha Vrksasana

1. Squat down. Place the hands, palms down and shoulder–width apart, on the floor in front of you, 6 inches (15 cm) from the wall.

2. Raise the hips, straighten the arms, and begin to bring the body weight into the hands. Inhale and on an exhale, kick the right leg up toward the wall followed by the left. Push up from the palms, straighten the elbows, and lift the shoulders and chest. Tuck the tailbone in to reduce the arch in the back. Bring the feet together, make the legs strong, and extend the heels upward. Breathe 8 or more times and come down by dropping one leg toward the floor. Return to a squatting position for a few minutes before standing.

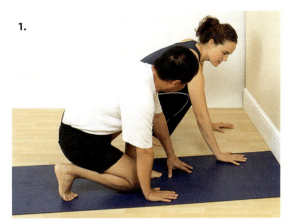

1.

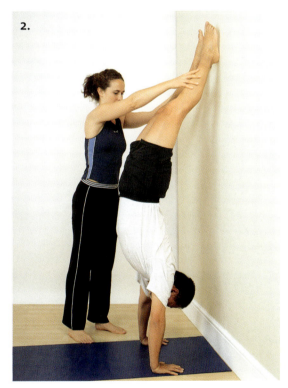

2.

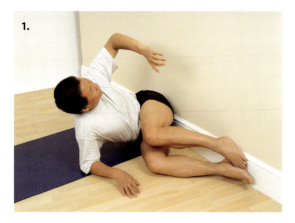

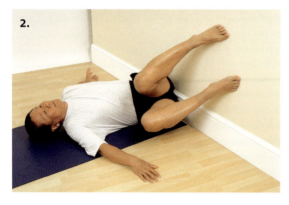

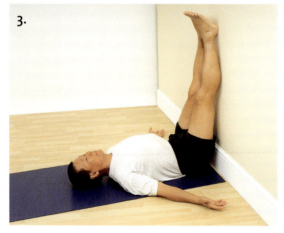

Legs up the wall *Viparita Karani*

1. Sit sideways and shift the buttocks close to the wall, with the left hip pointing up.

2. Once the buttocks are in place, release the side of the torso to the floor, roll over onto the back, and raise the legs up the wall.

3. Straighten through the backs of the legs, so that the backs are touching the wall. Tuck the chin in slightly and lengthen through the back of the neck. Flex the feet and extend through the backs of the legs. Relax the arms alongside the body. Hold for 10 to 15 minutes.

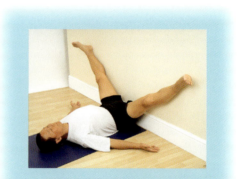

✴ **TIP** To stretch the inside of the legs and to create flexibility in the hips, practice the pose with the legs apart.

Half-moon pose *Ardha Chandrasana*

1. Stand with your back against a wall with the feet 3 to 4 feet (1 to 1.2 m) apart. Turn the right leg and foot out toward the end of the mat and turn the back foot in slightly. Extend the arms out to the sides. Inhale, and on an exhalation bend the right leg and place the fingertips of the right hand on the floor or on a block about 1.5 feet (just over a meter) in front of the right foot. Draw the back foot in slightly. At the same time, straighten the right leg and lift the left leg up until it is parallel with the floor.

2. Extend the left arm so that both arms form a straight line against the wall. Keep rotating the chest and lifting the left hip so that the body is on one plane. Stretch into the heel of the left leg. Turn the head to look up toward the left thumb. Maintain the weight in the standing leg, not the arm. Breathe steadily for 8 breaths. Repeat the pose on the other side.

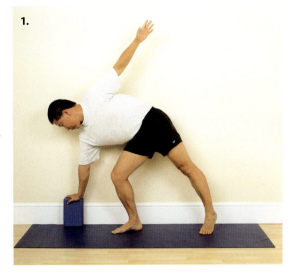

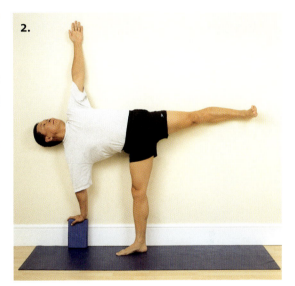

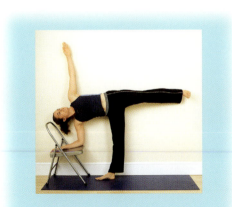

✳ **TIP** To make the pose even more accessible, practice the pose using a chair for additional height and support.

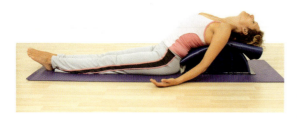

Opening the upper chest and neck

Sit in *dandasana* (see page 79) with your bottom at the base of the arch. Gently lower yourself backward onto the arch. Now relax the head and neck, soften the shoulders and open the chest. Focus on opening up the heart center, or chakra, in the chest. Breathe steadily and evenly for 10 minutes.

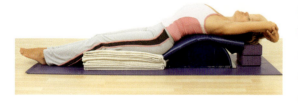

Opening the thorax, spine, and side ribs

Place 3 or 4 folded blankets at the base of the back arch and two blocks at the back of the arch. Sit in *dandasana* (see page 79) at the base of the arch. Gently lower yourself backward over the back arch, allowing the back of the head to be supported by the blocks. Extend the arms over the head and take hold of opposite elbows. Enjoy the stretch, breathing easily for 5 to 10 minutes.

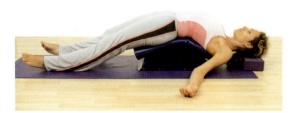

Opening the lower back and pelvis

Sit part way up the back arch, then gently lower yourself backward over the arch. Place a block under the back of the head for additional support. Extend the legs away. Allow the arms to fall naturally to the sides with the palms facing up. Relax for 10 to 15 minutes.

✳ **TIP** Depending upon where you lie on the arch (see also page 26) the back arch will stretch a different part of the back. Made from molded plastic, a back arch can feel hard, slippery, and generally uncomfortable without padding, so it is advisable to place it on top of a sticky mat and then fold a second sticky mat over the arch for additional support. Detailed here are four variations using the back arch. Some of the exercises use blocks and blankets (see pages 26, 27) which (as with all poses) you should place within easy reach of your mat before you begin.

Half-shoulder stand with a back arch

Sit on the top of the back arch. Gently lower yourself back over the arch until the shoulders are on the mat. Tuck the chin in and extend through the back of the neck. Lift the legs up into a vertical position, one leg at a time. Place the hands on the floor with palms facing down-ward, alongside the arch. Relax for 5 minutes, breathing evenly.

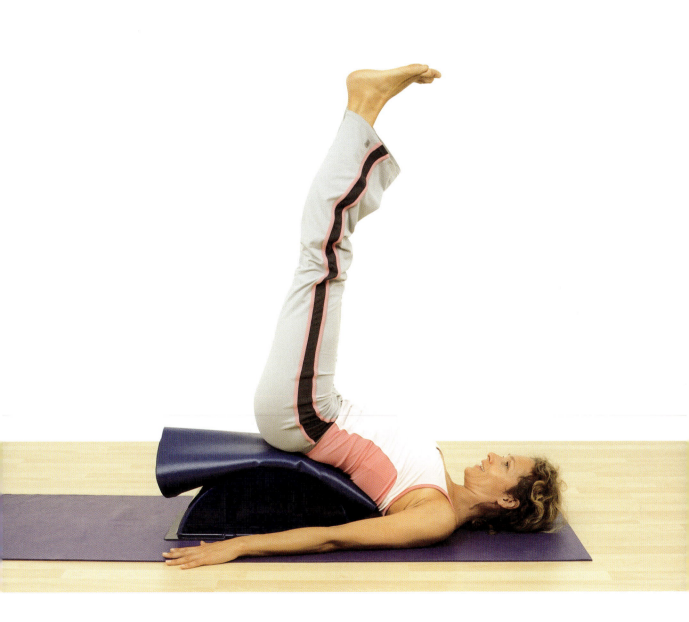

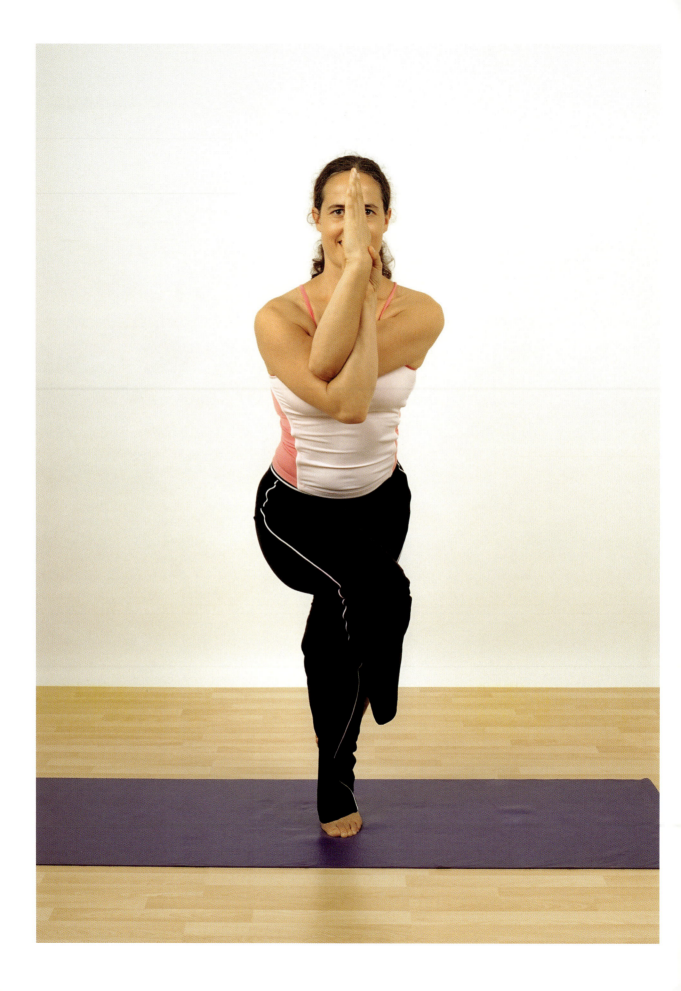

CHAPTER 2

Maintaining Healthy Joints

Warm-up stretches help to loosen the 12 primary joints in the body—both ankles, knees, hips, wrists, elbow, and shoulders, as well as warm the spine. The exercises are useful for anyone suffering from arthritis or recovering from injury. The warm-up series releases residual tension in the muscles, eases stiffness in the joints, and prepares the body for the more complex poses. On a subtle level, they also remove energy blocks, allowing prana, or energy, to move smoothly around the body, giving greater freedom of movement. It is important to perform the warm-up exercises gently and without strain, following the natural rotation of the joint. While practicing the movements, bring awareness to the interaction of the joints, ligaments, and muscles, and observe how each movement relates to other areas of the body.

Neck side stretch

Stand in *tadasana* (see page 60), or sit upright on a supportive chair. Bend and lift the right elbow and place the right hand on the left side of the head, with the elbow pointing to the side as shown. Inhale. Exhale, gently pulling the head to the right toward the right shoulder. Keep the head facing forward, and make sure that the left shoulder stays relaxed and down. Hold the position for a few seconds, breathing evenly, then repeat it on the opposite side.

BENEFITS   The neck movements tone all the nerves that pass through the neck and are connected to the different parts of the body. Practicing them can help relieve stiffness and tension from the neck and shoulders.

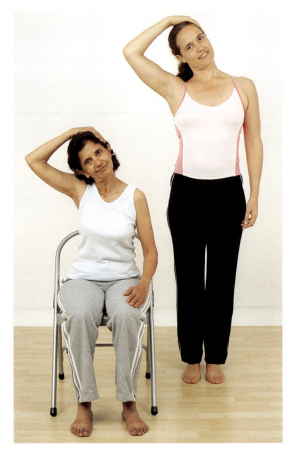

Head turns

1. Stand in *tadasana* (see page 60) or sit upright on a chair, and inhale. Exhale and turn the head to look over the left shoulder. Hold for a few moments, breathing evenly.

2. Inhale, turn back to the center and repeat on the other side.

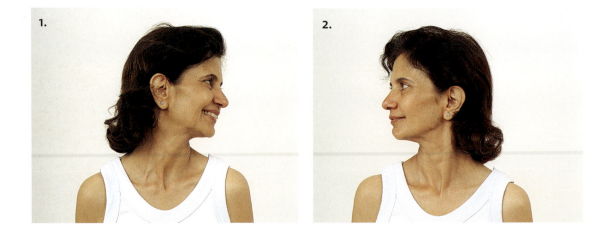

Head rolls

1. Practice the steps of this asana as one flowing movement. Begin by standing or sitting upright in a comfortable seated position, with the arms and shoulders relaxed. On an exhalation, lower the chin toward the sternum.

2. On an inhalation, gently roll the head up and to the side to look over the right shoulder. Make the movement as soft and fluid as possible. Continue to roll the head up on the inhalation to look up toward the ceiling. Make sure that the shoulder blades relax down the back.

3. Exhale, slowly drop the head to the opposite side to look over the left shoulder, then roll the head back to the first position. Repeat the exercise twice in each direction. If you feel discomfort in the neck, rest in that position for a moment or two and breathe into the area to release the tension.

1.
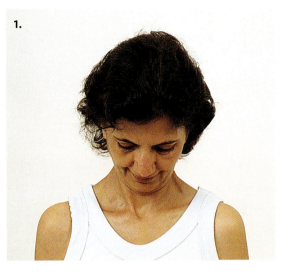

2.
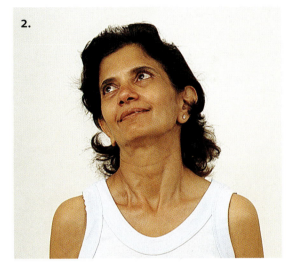

3.
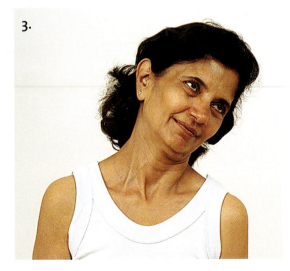

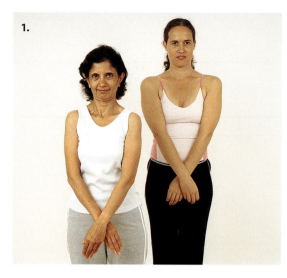

Shoulder circles

1. Stand in *tadasana* (see page 60) with the feet together. Make loose fists with the hands and cross the arms at the wrists.

2. Inhale and slowly rotate the arms up and over the head. Make sure that the shoulders stay relaxed.

3. Continue the rotation on an exhalation, allowing the arms to naturally move out to the sides. Rotate the arms back and out to the sides, moving all the way around and back to the starting position. Repeat the rotation at least twice in one direction, and then twice in the opposite direction. When you circle the shoulders in the opposite direction, rotate the arms backward and cross the wrists above the head to come forward.

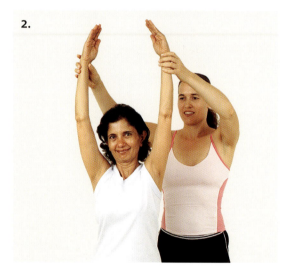

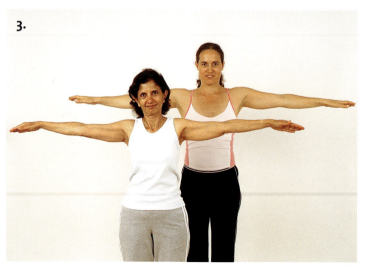

Elbow bends

1. Stand or sit upright in a comfortable seated position, with the arms and shoulders relaxed. Inhale, bend the elbows and place the hands or fingertips on the shoulders.

2. Exhale, straighten the elbows, and extend the arms forward. Repeat 3 to 5 times.

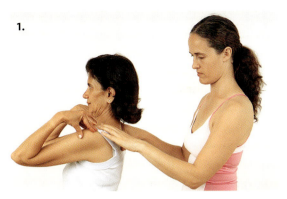

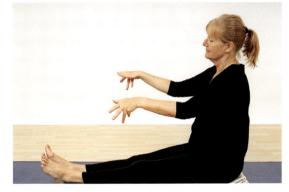

Wrist rotations

Stand or sit upright in a comfortable seated position, with the arms and shoulders relaxed. Lift the arms to an easy position and gently rotate the hands in a circular motion, 10 times in one direction and then 10 times in the opposite direction.

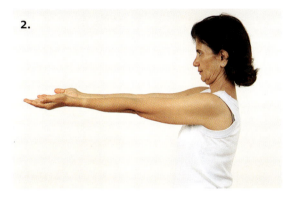

Ankle rolls

Sit in *dandasana* (see page 79) with the legs outstretched. Lift the right leg a few inches from the floor and gently circle the foot, holding the leg as shown. Rotate 10 times in one direction and then 10 times in the opposite direction. Repeat with the other leg.

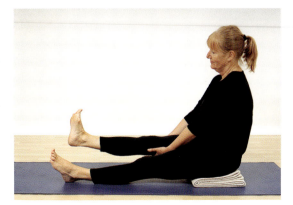

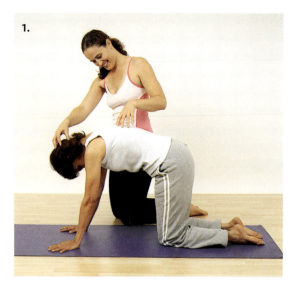

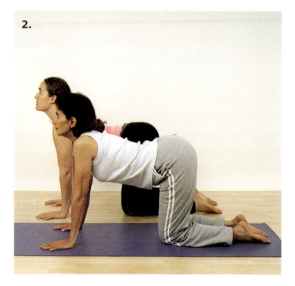

Cat pose *Majariasana*

This pose warms and limbers the whole spine. Initiate movement from the base of the spine.

1. Start on all fours, with hands beneath the shoulders and the knees beneath the hips. Inhale, lift the tailbone, concave the spine, and drop the belly. Press the hands into the floor, lift the chest and head, and look up.

2. Exhale, tuck the tailbone under, arch the back, and roll your head under, moving the chin toward the chest. Stretch the spine as high as you can. Curl the tailbone under. Repeat steps 1 and 2 for a few rounds. Make the movements as fluid as possible in time with the breath.

Eagle pose *Garudasana*

1. Stand in *tadasana* (see page 60). Focus on a spot in front of you for balance. Inhale, and raise the arms over the head.

2. Exhale as you release your arms, passing the right arm under the left arm.

3. Twist the arms around each other and touch palms. Bend the elbows so the palms are in front of the nose. Inhale.

4. Exhale, bend the knees and lift the right thigh over the left thigh. Wrap the right foot around the left calf. Try to keep knees and elbows in one line in the center of the body. Hold for 8 seconds, breathing evenly. Release and repeat on the opposite side.

BENEFITS   Eagle pose strengthens the ankles and calves, removes stiffness in the hips and shoulders, improves circulation, and develops concentration and balance.

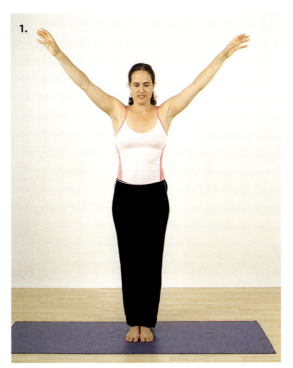

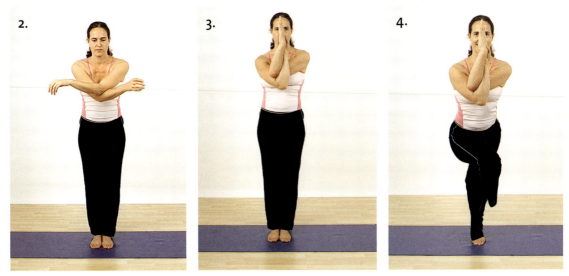

Sun salutation *Surya Namaskar*

Surya Namaskar is a dynamic series of 14 asanas that are linked together with the breath. The flow of asana acts as a complete body warm-up that creates heat in the body, which limbers the spine and tones the joints, muscles, and internal organs.

1. Stand in *tadasana* (see page 60) at the front of the mat with the feet together, and the palms touching in front of the chest.

2. Inhale and stretch the arms up over the head and look toward the thumbs. Lift the chest up and gently arch the back. Keep the arms along-side the ears. Be careful not to strain the lower back.

3. Exhale and bend forward from the hips, keeping the back and legs straight and the arms extended.

4. Bend the head down toward the knees and place the hands on either side of the feet. If the hands do not touch the floor, bend the knees.

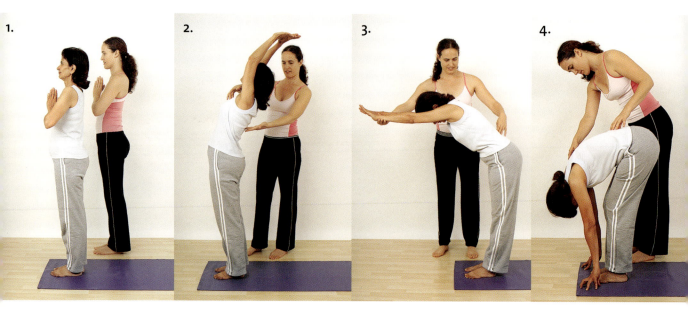

1. 2. 3. 4.

5. Inhale and stretch the right leg far back and drop the right knee to the floor. Lift the chest, and look up.

6. Exhale and step the left foot in line with the right. Come into a downward-facing dog by pushing into the hands, lifting the pelvis up and back, and stretching the heels toward the floor. Relax the head and neck and look toward the feet. Inhale.

7. Exhale, bend the knees to the floor and the elbows backward; lower the chest to the floor, leaving the pelvis raised. Place the chin on the floor.

8. Inhale, drop the pelvis, tuck the tailbone under and slide the body forward, lengthening the spine. Lift the head, neck, and chest without too much pressure in the hands. Look up. Keep the pelvis on the floor.

5.

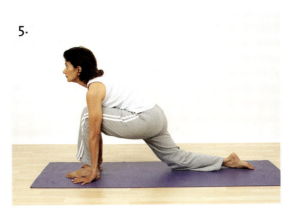

6.

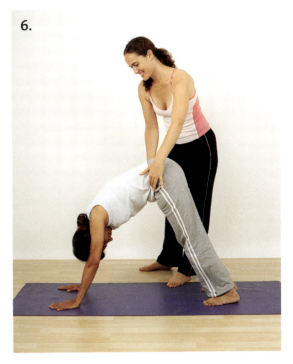

7.

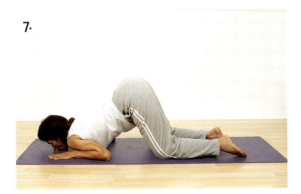

8.

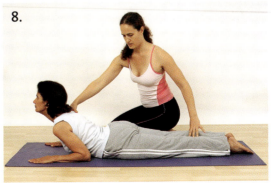

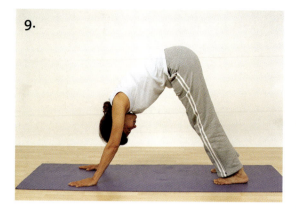

9. Exhale and push into the hands, raising the buttocks and back into downward dog pose, so that the body forms a triangle. Relax the crown of the head toward the floor and release the neck. Keep lengthening the spine and take the heels to the floor.

10. Inhale, step the right foot forward, in line with the hands. Lower the right knee to the floor, lift the chest, lengthen the spine, and look up.

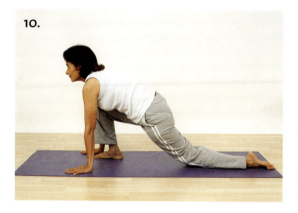

11. Exhale. Step the left foot forward in line with the right foot, coming into a forward bend. Lift up the pelvis and straighten through the backs of the knees. Relax the head toward the knees.

12. Inhale, stretch the arms forward alongside the ears, elongate the spine, lift the torso, and return to standing with the arms raised over the head.

13. Lift the chest and gently arch the back.

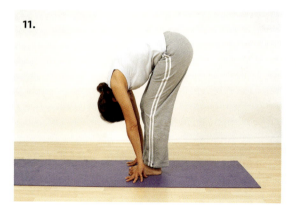

14. Exhale and bring the hands into prayer position in front of the chest. Repeat the cycle leading with the left foot to complete one full round of *Surya Namaskar.*

12. **13.** **14.**

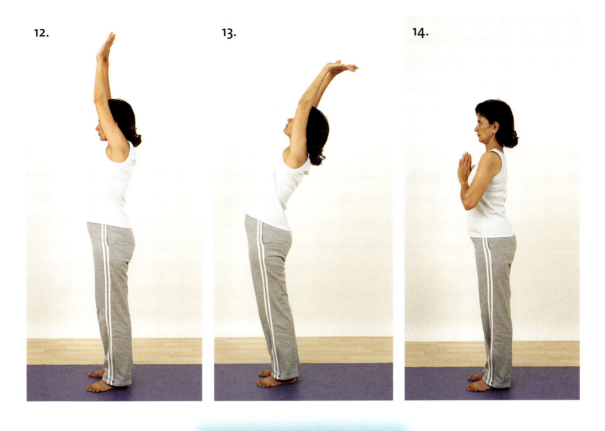

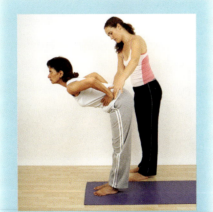

✳ **TIP** If you are suffering from a lower back problem then bend the knees and place the hands on the hips to move in and out of the forward bends, steps 4 and 12.

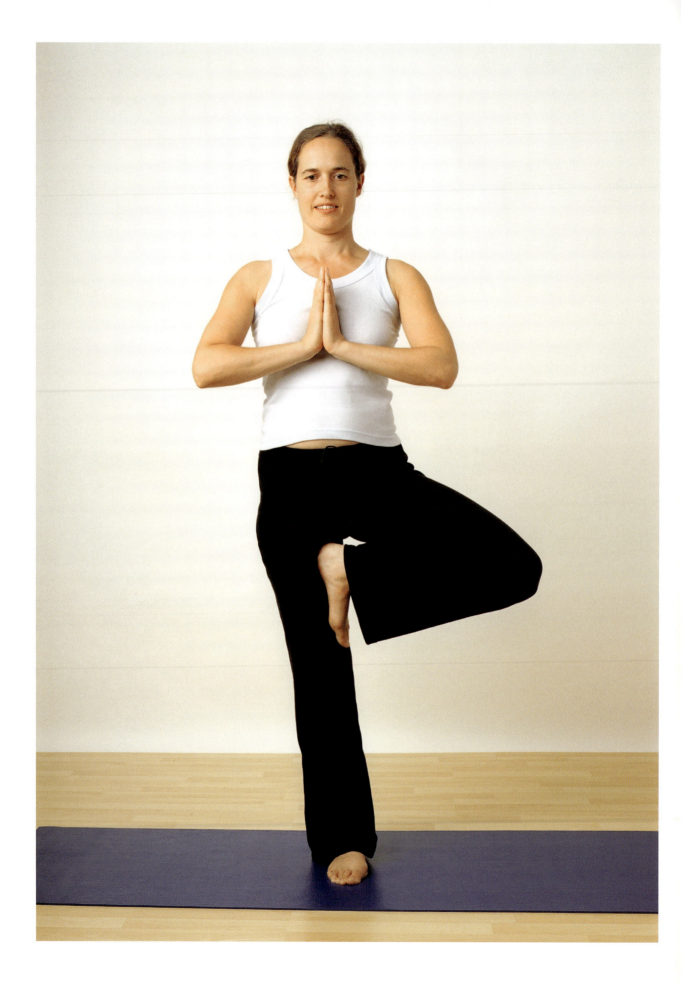

CHAPTER 3

Standing Poses

The standing poses help to build a strong and stable foundation starting from the feet upward, as well as improving balance and coordination. More importantly, they teach us to stand on our own two feet, building confidence, poise, and grace. A refreshing tonic for the entire body, standing poses stimulate breathing, improve the circulation, aid the digestive system, and improve our mobility; they are particularly beneficial for those suffering from arthritis and rheumatism. Standing poses act as further warm-up exercises because they warm the larger muscle groups of the body with their larger movements. Due to the rotational and bending motion of the standing poses, the major joints of the body are lubricated and the skeletal structure is realigned. For safety, remember always to practice these poses on a non-slip surface.

Mountain pose *Tadasana*

Tadasana is the primary standing pose that teaches realignment and balance, and steadies the mind. Return to tadasana between each standing pose.

1. Stand with the feet together and spread the toes. Stand straight, with the spine elongated and the chest lifted. Distribute the weight evenly on both feet. Keep the legs strong and lift the knees up by pulling up the thigh muscles. The head, shoulders, and hips should be directly over the ankles with the tailbone tucked under slightly. Keep the arms extended along the sides of the body, with the hands relaxed.

2. Roll the shoulders forward and back, so the shoulder blades relax down the back. Tuck the chin in slightly, extending the back of the neck. Feel the lower half of the body from the navel down rooted into the ground, and feel the upper body from the navel up lifting toward the heavens. Breathe evenly for 8 or more breaths.

1.

2.

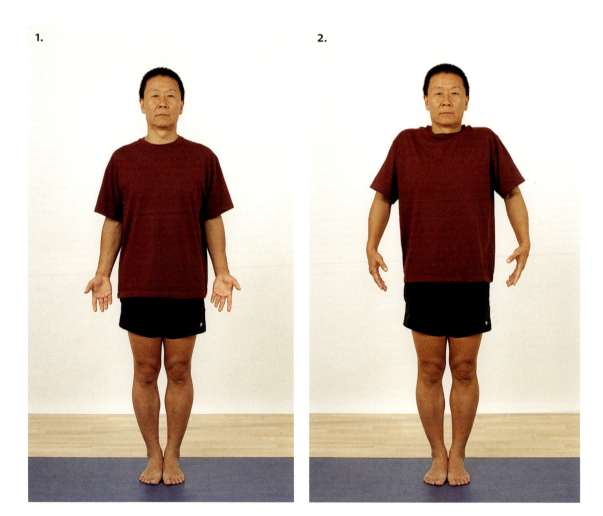

Raised-arm mountain pose

Urdhva Hastasana

1. Stand in *tadasana* (see opposite). Inhale and extend the arms out to the sides and up until the arms are parallel overhead.

2. Straighten through the elbows and look up. Breathe evenly for 8 breaths. Release the arms.

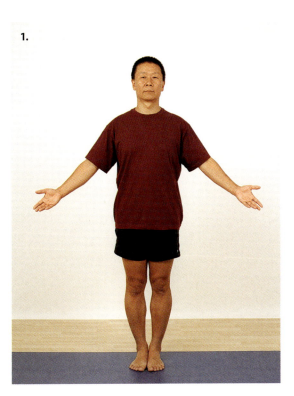

1.

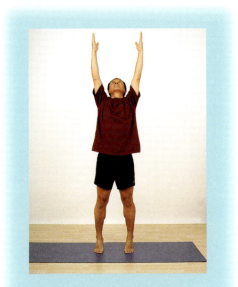

✳ **TIP** This variation helps to stretch and strengthen the toes. Stand with the feet hip-width apart. Inhale and raise the arms overhead. Push down through the balls of the feet and rise up on to tiptoes. Stretch up for 8 breaths.

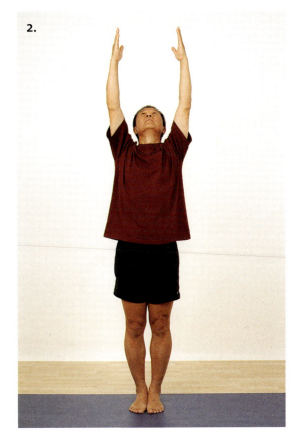

2.

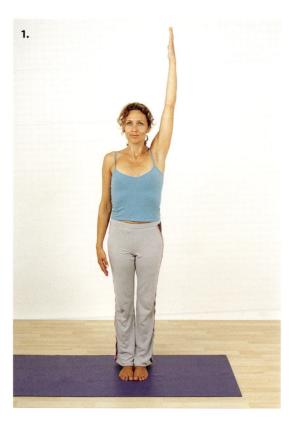

1.

Standing side stretch *Tiryaka Tadasana*

1. Stand in *tadasana* (see page 60). Inhale and raise the left arm up, alongside the head, with the palm facing toward you.

2. Exhale, pushing the hips over to the left, lift up out of the waist and stretch the body over to the right. Feel the stretch along the left side from the heels to the toes. Do not collapse on the right side. Hold for 8 breaths. Repeat on the opposite side.

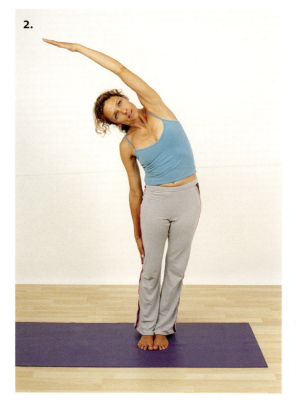

2.

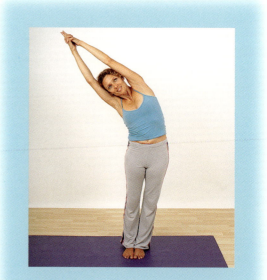

✳ **TIP** For a more intense stretch raise both arms overhead, interlock the fingers, except for the index fingers, and repeat the above exercise

Forward bend 1 *Uttanasana I*

1. Stand with the feet together and inhale. Place the hands on the hips and lift the chest. Exhale and bend forward as far as possible without bending the knees.

2. Clasp behind the ankles and draw the face to the knees with the hips in line with the feet. Lift up the inner arches of the feet, keep the legs strong, and relax the upper body. Hold for 8 breaths.

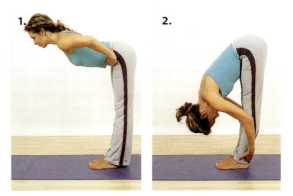

Forward bend 2 *Uttanasana II*

This variation releases tension in the neck and shoulders.

1. Stand with the feet together and inhale. If you have lower back pain, practice this pose with the toes turned in slightly. Clasp the hands behind the back, stretch the shoulder blades down, and lift the hands away from the buttocks.

2. Exhale. Leading with the chest, bend forward from the hips and take the head toward the knees. Soften the shoulders, release the arms, and stretch the hands away.

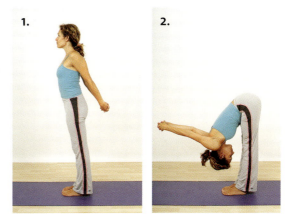

BENEFITS   In forward bend, the heart is rested and the organs of the head receive a fresh suply of oxygen-rich blood.

✳ **VARIATION**   To learn to bend forward with a straight back, stand with the feet hip-width apart. Bend forward and place the hands on the back of a chair. In this position, focus on lengthening the spine by lifting through the backs of the legs and stretching the pelvis back away from the head.

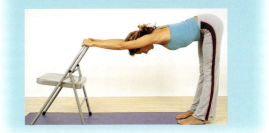

Powerful pose *Utkatasana*

Stand in *tadasana* (see page 60) with the feet hip-width apart and the outside edges of the feet parallel. Inhale and raise the arms to shoulder height, palms facing the floor. Exhale and bend the legs, as if you were going to sit down on a chair. Keep the legs parallel, shift the body weight into the heels and lift the chest. Hold for 8 breaths.

BENEFITS *Utkatasana*, powerful pose, strengthens the ankles, knees, and thighs, and shapes the legs. It reduces stiffness in the back and tones the spine.

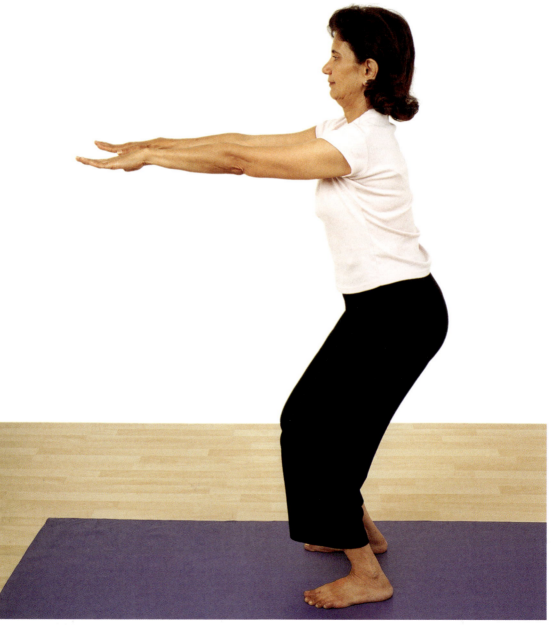

Triangle pose *Trikonasana*

1. Stand with the feet 3 to 4 feet (1 to 1.2 m) apart with the arms extended at shoulder height with the palms facing the floor. Relax the shoulders and pull the kneecaps up by tightening the thigh muscles. Turn the right leg out so that the right foot points toward the end of the mat, keeping the knee in line with the ankle. Turn the left foot in slightly toward the right side, the instep in line with the right heel.

2. Inhale and on exhalation bend to the right, placing the right hand on the ankle or as far down the leg as you can reach. Stretch the left arm up and turn the head to look up. Keep the left hip lifted and rotate the chest so that the body is in one plane. Breathe steadily for 8 breaths. Repeat on the left side.

BENEFITS *Trikonasana* improves flexibility in the spine, and alleviates back and neck pain. It massages and tones the pelvis and abdomen, relieving indigestion and gas.

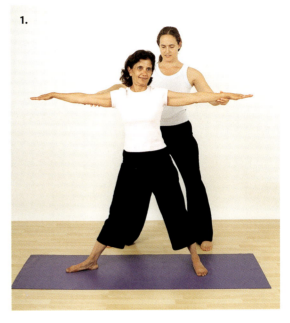

1.

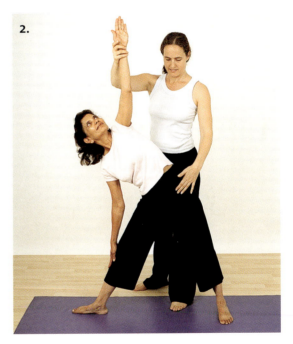

2.

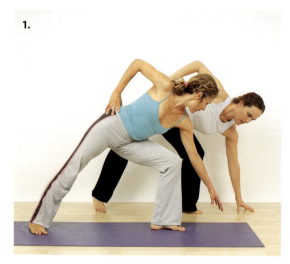

Half-moon pose *Ardha Chandrasana*

1. Step the feet 3 to 4 feet (1 to 1.2 m) apart. Turn the left leg and foot out toward the end of the mat and turn the back foot in slightly. Place the right hand on the right hip. Exhale, bend the left knee and bend sideways, placing the hand on the floor about 1 foot (30 cm) from the front foot. Inhale.

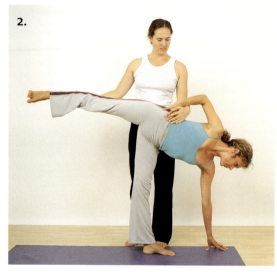

2. Exhale and draw the back foot in, straighten the left leg and lift the right leg up until it is parallel with the floor. Rotate the chest and lift the right hip so that the body is on one plane.

3. Extend the right arm so that both arms form a straight line. Stretch into the heel of the left leg and look up at the right thumb. Maintain the weight in the standing leg, not the arm. Breathe steadily 8 or more times, then repeat the pose on the other side.

BENEFITS *Ardha chandrasana*, improves concentration and balance, bringing agility and lightness to the body, and relieves backache and sciatica. The pose helps to correct a prolapsed uterus.

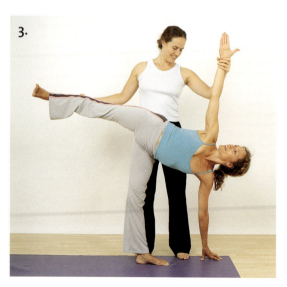

Extended side stretch *Parsvakonasana*

1. Step the feet 4 to 4½ feet (1.2 to 1.4 m) apart. Extend the arms out to the sides. Rotate the right leg and foot 90 degrees, but keep the hips facing forward and turn in the left foot slightly. Bend the right knee until it is directly over the ankle joint.

2. Inhale, then on an exhalation lean over to the right side, and place the right hand on the outside of the right foot with fingers in line with the toes. Keep the feet grounded and maintain pressure along the outside edge of the left foot. Keep the thigh of the bent leg parallel to the edge of the mat and the knee at a right angle. Rotate the left arm until the palm is facing up, then extend it alongside the left ear, forming a diagonal line along the left side of the body from the heel to the fingertips. Turn the head and look up. Breathe evenly for 8 breaths. Repeat the pose on the opposite side.

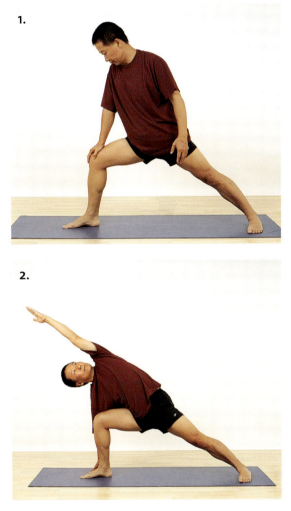

1.

2.

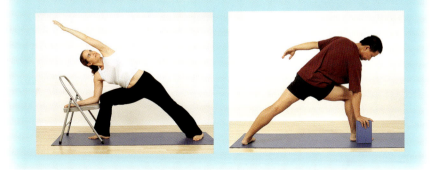

✳ **TIP** Practice the pose using a chair or a brick for support. Place a chair in front of the right knee, lean the body to the right and place the right forearm on the chair seat. alternatively rest your hand on a brick by your outside ankle.

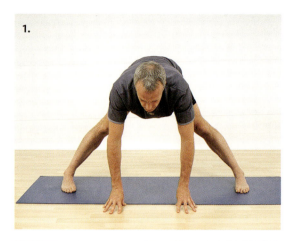

Extended leg pose *Padottanasana*

1. Step the feet 4 to 4½ feet (1.2 to 1.4 m) apart and place the hands on the hips. With the feet parallel and the legs strong, bend forward with a flat back, placing the hands on the floor directly under the shoulders. Keep the hips in line with the heels and extend the torso from the pelvis to the crown of the head. Breathe 8 times.

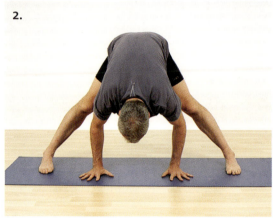

2. Exhale, walk the hands in line with the feet. Take the head toward the floor between the hands. Relax the body and keep the legs strong. Maintain the pose for 8 breaths.

✳ **TIP** For beginners, place the hands on blocks in Step 2 and focus on elongating the spine.

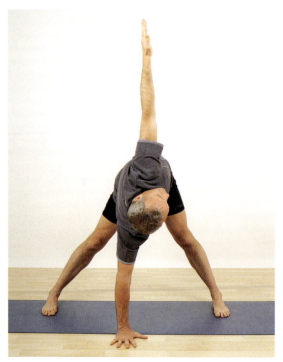

Extended leg pose twist

Parivrtta Padottanasana

Step the feet 4 to 4½ feet (1.2 to 1.4 m) apart and place the hands on the hips. Keep the feet parallel and the legs strong. Bend forward with a flat back and place the right hand on the floor, centered between your legs. Raise the left arm and rotate the chest to the left. Look up toward the raised hand. Hold for 8 breaths, then return to the center and repeat on the opposite side.

Sideways extended pose

Parsvottanasana

1. Step the feet 3½ feet (1 m or so) apart, placing the right foot forward. Turn the right foot and leg toward the end of the mat.

Lift up onto the ball of the left foot and turn the left foot in line with the right. Rotate the hips to face forward. Place the hands on the hips and extend the spine, and inhale.

2. Exhale and extend forward over the right leg. Place the hands down on the floor alongside the right leg. Bend the head toward the right leg. Hold for 8 breaths. Repeat on the opposite side.

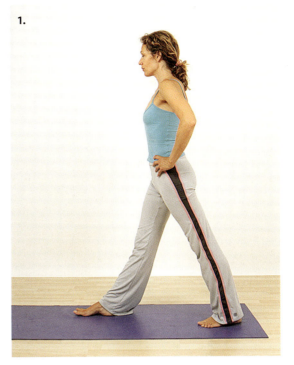

1.

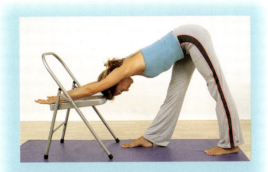

✳ **TIP** If you have difficulty bending to the floor, you can use a chair to help with this exercise.

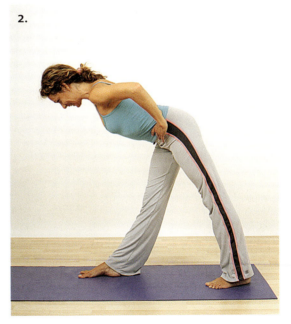

2.

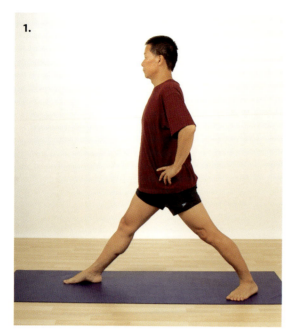

1.

Warrior pose 1 *Virabhadrasana I*

1. Step the feet 4 to 4½ feet (1.2 to 1.4 m) apart. Place the hands on the hips and then turn both feet and the hips to the right, to face the end of the mat. Inhale.

2. Raise the arms over the head into prayer position. Bend the right knee to form a right angle, lift the chest and look up. Hold for 8 breaths. Repeat on the opposite side.

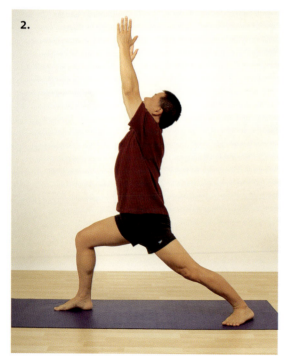

2.

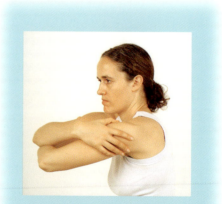

✳ **TIP** As a counter stretch to Warrior 2 (a stretch in the opposite direction to the muscles worked in the pose) place the hands on the opposite shoulders and stretch into the back between the shoulder blades.

Warrior pose 2 *Virabhadrasana II*

1. Step the feet 4 to 4½ feet (1.2 to 1.4 m) apart. Turn the right foot and leg to face the end of the mat and turn the left foot in. Extend the arms at shoulder height with palms down. Inhale.

2. Exhale. Bend the right knee to form a right angle, with the knee directly over the ankle. Keep the torso upright, and turn the head to look over the right shoulder.

3. Hold the pose for 8 breaths, then repeat on the opposite side.

1.

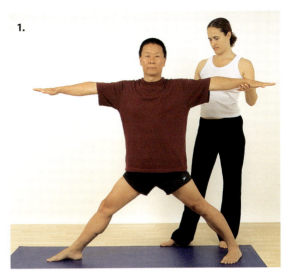

2.

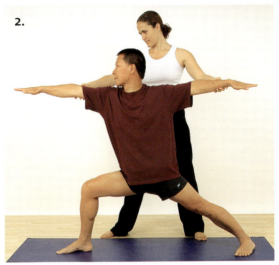

3.

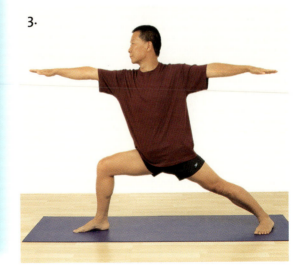

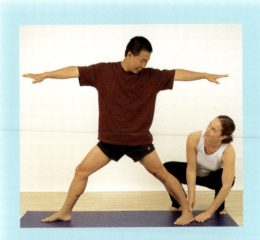

✳ **TIP** Check the position of the non-leading foot, ensuring that it stays turned inward as you move through the pose.

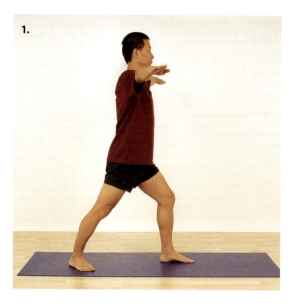

1.

Warrior pose 3 *Virabhadrasana III*

1. Stand at the end of the mat. Inhale and extend and lift the arms out to the sides. Step forward with the left leg, lean forward, and as you do this shift the body weight into the left leg.

2. Now exhale and simultaneously lift up the right leg and the back to form a straight line running from the crown of the head to the toes. Keep the hips on one plane and the head in line with the spine. Breathe 8 times, then repeat the pose on the opposite side.

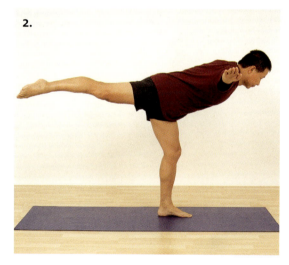

2.

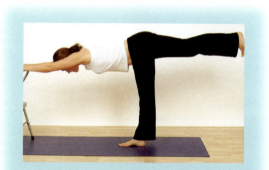

✳ **TIP** Try this pose using a chair for support. Place a chair with the back toward you about 4 feet (1.2 m) in front. (Make sure that the chair is placed on the mat as shown, or against a wall, so that it will not slip.) Bend forward and place the hands on top of the back of the chair. Raise the right leg up until it is parallel to the floor. Keep the hips level, in line with the raised leg. Hold for 8 breaths. Repeat on the opposite side.

Tree pose *Vrksasana*

Stand in tadasana *(see page 60) and spread the toes. Begin to take the body weight into the left leg.*

Raise the right leg and place the sole of the foot on the inside of the left thigh, pressing the muscle of the right leg against the left foot for support. Bring the palms together in front of the chest.

Hold for 8 breaths. To help with balance, pick a spot to concentrate on, either on the wall or about 4 feet (1.2 m) in front on the floor, or practice the pose with your back against the wall. Keep the breathing smooth and steady.

If you find that it is difficult to raise the leg as far as the inner thigh, place it either on the stationary foot or on the inside of the stationary knee. Use a chair or a wall for additional support.

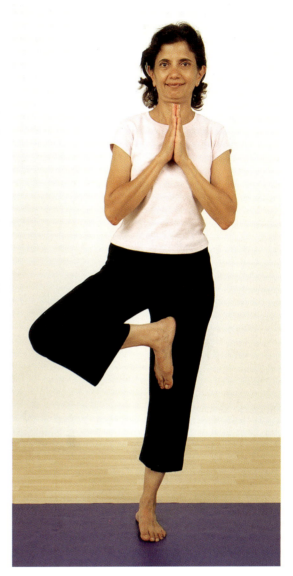

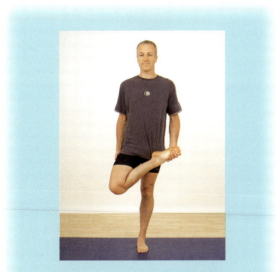

✳ **TIP** For an increases hip stretch bend the right leg and place the right ankle on top of the left thigh. Hold the right foot and rotate the right knee toward the floor. Hold for 8 breaths. repeat on the opposite side.

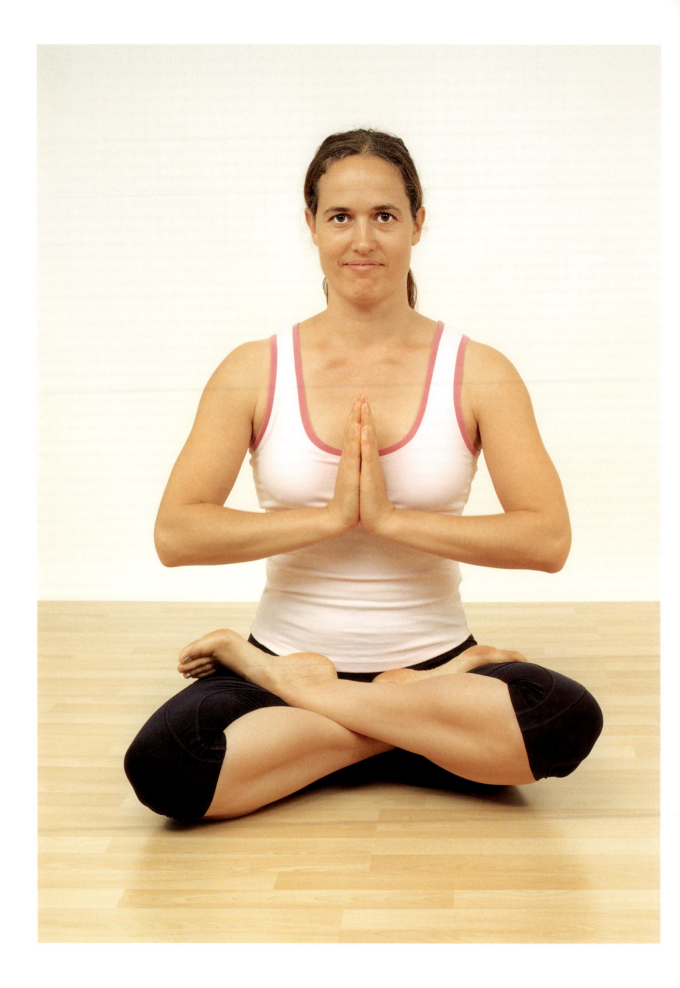

CHAPTER 4

Hip Openers

Falling is one of the greatest risks in later life, although older people who keep mobile are less likely to fall. The hip, which is essentially a ball-and-socket joint, is the largest joint in the body. Maintaining flexibility in the hips is key to remaining mobile. The following poses flex and open the hip joint. The forward bends also provide traction, creating space between the vertebrae of the spine, supplying a fresh supply of oxygen and blood to the discs, and toning the back. The following poses are suitable to practice during menstruation and menopause, and they also help regulate hormone production. Do not strain in the poses; relaxation is the key to their accomplishment.

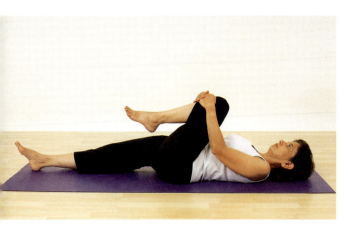

One knee to chest

Ardha Supta Pawanmuktaasana

Lie on your back with the feet together. Raise the left leg and bend the knee. Interlock the fingers around the shin. Inhale and on an exhalation, hug the bent leg close to the chest. Try to work the tailbone down toward the floor. Relax the head and neck and make sure that there is no tension in the jaw. Breathe 8 or more times. Repeat on the other side.

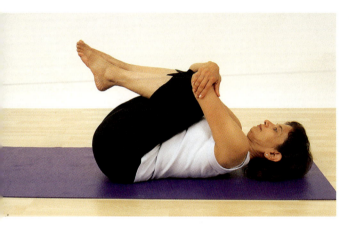

Both knees to chest

Supta Pawanmuktaasana

Lie on your back with the legs together. Bend both legs up toward the chest. Wrap the arms around the shins and on an exhalation, hug both knees closer in to the chest. As a counter stretch, curl the tailbone back down toward the floor. Keep the head and face relaxed. Hold for 8 breaths, then release the pose.

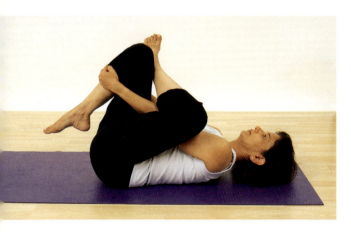

One knee to side

Supta Pawanmuktaasana

Lie on your back with the feet together. Bend both knees and place the feet on the floor close to the buttocks. Bend the left leg and place the ankle on top of the right thigh, just above the knee. Release the left knee out to the side. Reach through the inside of the left leg with the left hand and interlock the fingers around the right shin. Inhale, and on the exhalation pull the right knee in toward the chest. Hold for 8 breaths. Repeat on the opposite side.

Lying thumb-to-foot pose

Supta Padangushtasana

1. Lie flat on your back with the legs and feet together. Bend the left leg and take hold of the big toe with the thumb, index, and middle finger of the left hand.

2. Keeping hold of the big toe, inhale and straighten the left leg up, stretching into the heel of the left foot. Keep the left shoulder down, the hips level, and the right leg strong by pushing into the ground with the right thigh. Extend the right arm out to the side with the palm down.

3. Exhale and extend the left leg out to the left side, taking the heel toward the floor. Turn the head to look over the right shoulder. Hold for 8 breaths, then repeat on the opposite side.

BENEFITS As well as creating flexibility in the hips, *supta padangushtasana* is great for releasing tension and stiffness in the lower back. It tones the reproductive organs and stimulates the digestive tract.

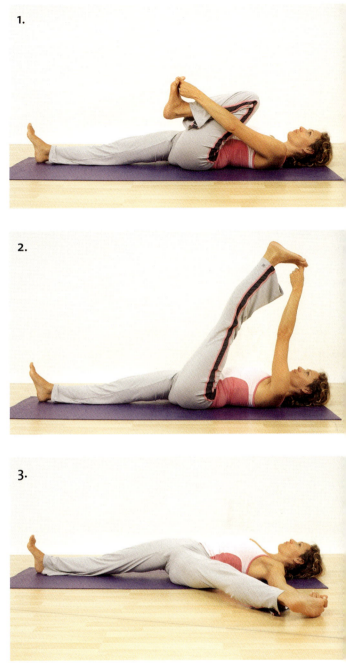

1.

2.

3.

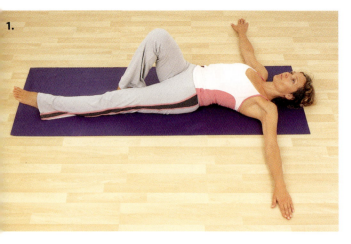

1.

Lying side stretch *Parivartanasana*

1. Lie on your back in a straight line. Extend the arms out to the side with the palms down. Bend the right knee and hook the right foot behind the left knee. Inhale.

2. Exhale and drop the right knee over to the left side. Keep both shoulders in contact with the mat. Look over the right shoulder. Relax the head, neck, and torso. Hold for 8 breaths, then repeat the pose on the opposite side.

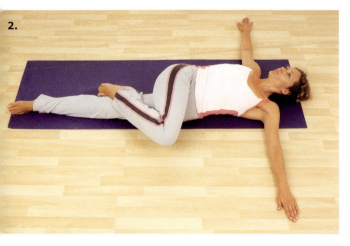

2.

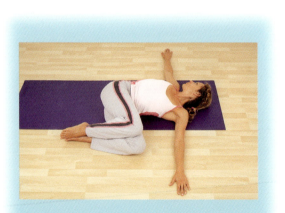

BENEFITS The twisting action of dropping the knees to the side massages and flexes the lower back, removing stiffness and tension.

✳ **TIP** For a more intense stretch, bend both knees up toward the chest. Stretch the arms out to the sides with the palms down on the floor. Inhale, then exhale and drop the knees over to the left side, revolving from the waist. Keep the right shoulder moving down toward the floor. Turn the head to look over to the right side. Relax the neck and release the back. Breathe evenly 8 or more times. Inhale, bring the legs to the center, then repeat on the other side.

Staff pose *Dandasana*

Sitting upright with the legs outstretched is called dandasana, *or staff pose. It is the neutral sitting pose for all forward bends, as is* tadasana *(see page 60) for standing poses. So between each sitting pose, come back to* dandasana.

Sit upright with the legs outstretched. Keep the ankles, knees, and thighs together. Extend through the backs of the legs into the heels and draw the toes toward the head. Keep the thighs strong and pressing down into the floor. Place the palms on the floor beside the hips with the fingers extending forward. Lift up the torso from the pelvic bones; draw the abdomen in toward the spine and up toward the diaphragm. Open the chest, lift the sternum, and move the shoulder blades back and down. Tuck the chin slightly in and lengthen through the back of the neck. Keep the head, shoulders, and hips in one line. Breathe steadily for 8 breaths.

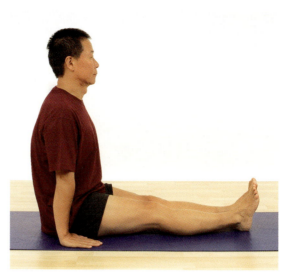

Hero pose *Virasana*

Kneel on the mat then lift the buttocks so that you are sitting on your knees. Keep the knees together and move the feet a little wider than hip-width apart, with the toes pointing backward. Slowly sit back down between the feet, easing the calf muscles out to the sides with the thumbs as you sit back. Sit up straight, lifting up from the pelvis. Hold for 8 breaths or longer, and then release.

> ✳ **TIP** If during this pose you experience any pain in your knees, or generally have difficulty sitting on the floor, take a folded blanket and place it between the feet, or rest a block under the buttocks.

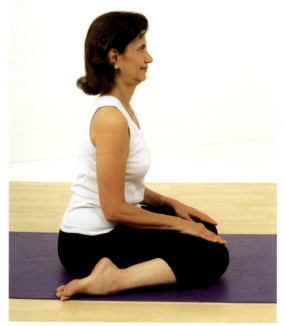

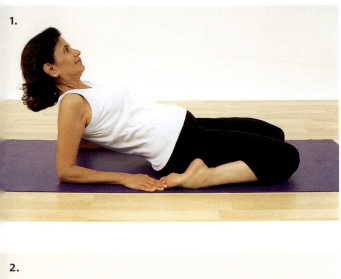

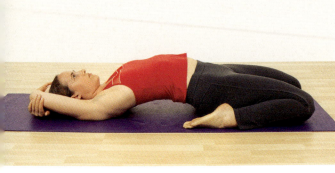

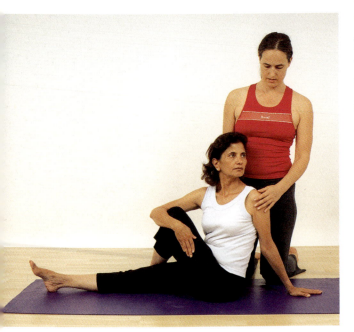

Lying hero pose *Supta Virasana*

1. When comfortable in *virasana* (see page 79) you can move on to *supta virasana*. Begin with *virasana*—inhale and exhale, reclining onto the elbows. Tuck the tailbone under. Feel the stretch through the front of the thighs and groin. Inhale, exhale, and take the upper back and head to the ground to continue the stretch.

2. Tuck the chin in slightly. Stretch the arms over the head and take hold of the elbows, stretching up from waist to elbows, opening the armpits, and down from the waist toward the kneecaps. Keep both sides of the body evenly extended. There should be no knee pain as the stretch is through the front of the body. Breathe evenly 8 or more times. exhale and slowly come up.

Sage pose *Marichyasana*

In *dandasana* (see page 79) bend the left knee, placing the foot outside the right knee. Lift and turn toward the bent leg, placing the left hand behind you on the floor. Press the right thigh into the floor, extending into the heel. Breathe in, exhale, and increase the twist; wrap the right arm around the left knee. Turn the torso and the head, looking over the left shoulder. Twist up from the base of the spine turning in the hips, waist, chest, and shoulders. Hold for 8 breaths, then repeat on other side.

Seated forward bend *Paschimottanasana*

Sit upright in *dandasana* (see page 79). Inhale. Stretch the arms up over the head and elongate the spine. Exhale, and bend forward with a flat back over your straight legs and take the hands to the sides of the feet or as far down the leg as possible. Take the elbows out to the sides and the head toward the knees. Relax the back of the neck and shoulders. Keep the legs straight, pressing the thighs in to the floor. Hold for 8 breaths, inhale, and come up.

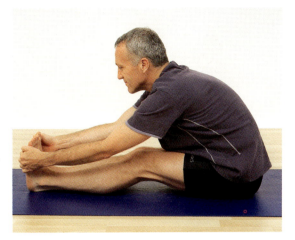

HAND VARIATIONS

Rather than touch the toes and lose a straight spine, hold the shins as you bend forward or, if you can reach the feet with a straight back, take hold of the big toes or the sides of the feet.

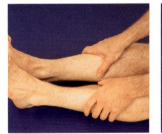
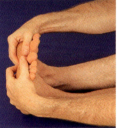

✳ **TIP** Building flexibility in the back and hamstrings requires patience and effort. If you cannot bend forward with a flat back and touch your feet, have a partner support your back or practice using a belt placed around the balls of the feet (see page 40). Only come as far forward as is comfortable without straining. As you bend forward, focus on keeping the spine erect and elongating the hamstrings.

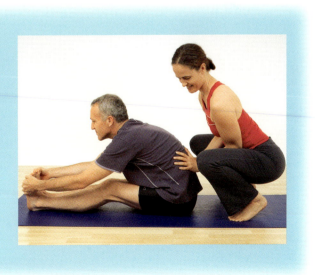

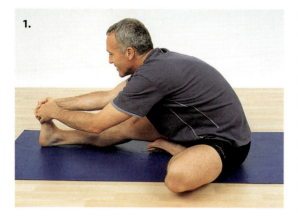

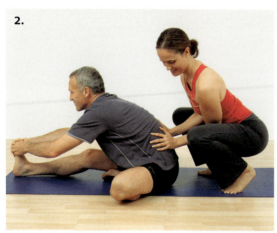

Head-to-knee pose *Janu Sirsasana*

1. Sit upright in *dandasana* (see page 79). Bend the left leg and place the sole of the left foot along the inside of the right thigh. Relax the left knee down to the floor. Keep the right leg strong and extend into the right heel. Inhale, elongate the spine and raise the arms over the head. Exhale, leading with the chest, and bend forward with a flat back over the extended leg. Hold the shin, ankle, or right foot with both hands. Bend the elbows to the side to gently pull deeper into the bend. Hold for 8 breaths. Repeat on the opposite side.

2. Keep your back flat and resist letting your spine curl. Ask a partner to assist you by supporting the lower back.

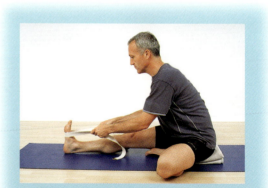

✳ **TIP** If you cannot reach the extended foot, use a belt around the ball of the extended foot (see page 40). Work on keeping the spine straight as you bend forward over the extended leg. Lift up and out of the lower back so that you pivot from the hip joints.

Rock the baby

1. Sit in *dandasana* (see page 79). Bend the right leg and take hold of the right ankle with both hands. Gently pull the ankle in and up, closer to the chest.

2. Place the right foot in the crook of the left arm, being careful to support the ankle joint. Wrap the right arm around the leg, placing the right knee in the crook of the right arm. Interlock the fingers around the outside of the right calf. Gently rock the right leg from side to side to open and massage the right hip joint. Continue rocking 8 to 10 times, breathing evenly. Repeat with the opposite leg.

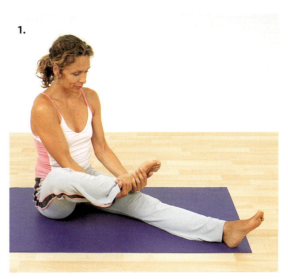

1.

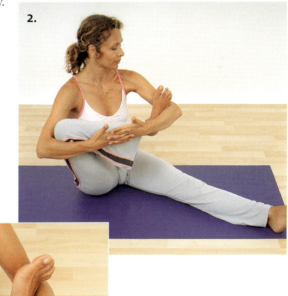

2.

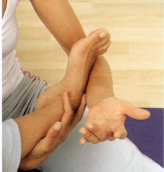

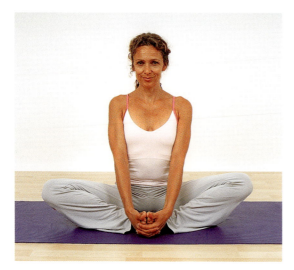

Cobbler pose *Baddha Konasana*

Sit in *dandasana* (see page 79) with the legs out-stretched. Bend both knees and bring the feet in as close to the groin as possible. Touch the soles of the feet together. Drop the knees to the sides. Hold the feet, keeping the spine straight and lifted. Hold for 8 breaths or longer.

BENEFITS *Baddha Konasana* is a gentle pose that increases mobility in the hip joint.

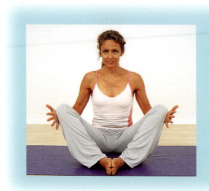

✳ **TIP** When coming out of the pose, support the knees with the hands and release slowly.

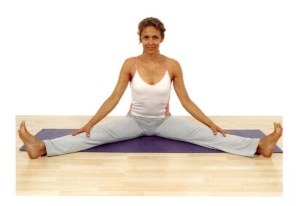

Seated angle pose *Upavista Konasana*

Sit in *dandasana* (see page 79). Stretch the legs out to the side as wide as possible. Keep the knees and feet pointing up. Press the thighs into the floor and extend into the heels. Place the hands on the legs, or the palms on the floor in front with fingers facing forward. Breathe evenly for 8 breaths.

✳ **TIP** The lower back has a tendency to sag or roll under in this pose. Place a block or folded blanket under the buttocks to lift the hips.

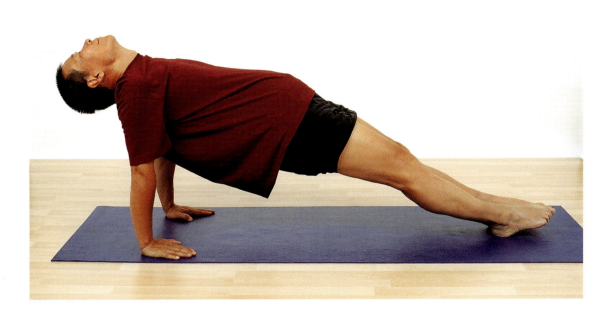

Table pose *Purvottanasana*

Purvottanasana provides the perfect counter-stretch to forward bending. It gently works the hips in the opposite direction, opens the groin, and releases tension in the lower back. Sit in *dandasana* (see page 79). Roll the shoulder blades toward the spine and to open the chest. Place the hands behind the back about 1 foot (30 cm) from the buttocks, with the fingers pointing forward. Inhale, lean into the hands, press down with both heels and lift the pelvis.

Point the toes and extend the soles of both feet onto the mat. Keep lifting up, open the chest, gently release the head and look back. Now exhale, then hold for 8 breaths, breathing evenly.

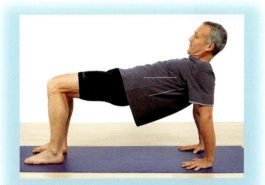

✳ **TIP** Sit in *dandasana* (see page 79). Place the hands behind the back about 1 foot (30 cm) from the buttocks. Bend the legs and place the soles of the feet on the mat, with the feet hip-width apart. Inhale, press into the hands and feet, and lift the pelvis and chest to form a horizontal line. Look forward toward the knees and hold for 8 breaths.

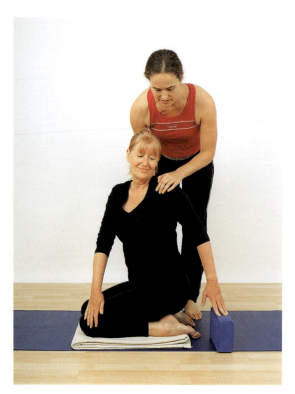

Gentle side twist

Come to a kneeling position. Inhale and extend the spine, keeping the hips, shoulders, and head in one line. Exhale, turn to the left and place the palm of the left hand on the outside of the right knee. Place the right hand on the floor or on a block behind the back. Look over the left shoulder. Keep twisting to the left, turning the navel, rib cage, shoulders and head. Breathe evenly for 8 breaths. Release the pose and repeat on the opposite side.

> ✳ **TIP** As you twist, do not allow the shoulders to lift—focus on keeping the shoulders relaxed and down.

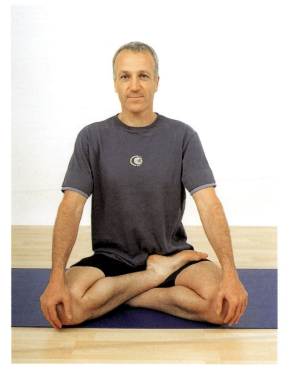

Half-lotus *Ardha Padmasana*

The half-lotus is a comfortable and safe seated pose that begins to open the hips in preparation for full lotus without straining the knees.

You can sit on a folded blanket or block to raise the hips and ease the lower back (see page 37). Sit in *dandasana* (see page 79). Bend your left leg and place the left foot close to the groin with the sole facing up. Bend the right leg and draw it close to both hands. Relax the right hip and leg completely. Lift the right foot and place it on top of the left thigh, with the sole facing upward. Sit straight with palms facing upward on your knees. Hold for 20 to 30 seconds. Release the legs and repeat on the opposite side.

Meditation

Meditation is an effective tool for managing stress because it helps to lower the level of cortisol, a hormone released by the adrenal glands in response to stress. Science has found a connection between stress and illness—when cortisol levels in the bloodstream remain too high for too long, disease can occur. Meditators have been found to have a much higher coping mechanism; they visit doctors and the hospital 50 percent less than non-meditators. The activity in the brain also changes during meditation as the brain waves become longer, akin to those produced during deeply relaxed states. The mind is gathered in the present, which cuts the natural tendency to worry about future events or obsess about previous actions. Also, meditation aids the circulation of blood to the brain, helping to keep the mind lucid in later life.

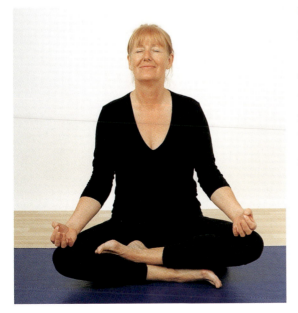

HOW TO MEDITATE

Meditation is usually practiced at the end of a yoga workout, after *pranayama* (see page 20). Like learning to play a musical instrument, meditation requires practice, for at least 20 minutes a day.

As a beginner it is important to find a peaceful spot in which to meditate that is free from external distractions such as ringing telephones or external street noise.

Find a comfortable position, either cross-legged, or in a half-lotus (see below left) or sitting on a chair with the spine upright. Wear loose-fitting, comfortable clothes and remove spectacles and watches.

It is important to maintain a passive attitude to any thoughts that arise in the mind, because initially when you sit the mind is flooded by all the activities of the day, from conversations that took place to lists of things you need to accomplish tomorrow.

Simply observe thoughts as if they were clouds floating across a clear blue sky and gently bring your awareness back to the breath or mantra. Observe the natural rhythm of your breathing, and the cool sensation as you breathe in and the warm sensation as you exhale. You can chant this mantra:

So Ham

So Ham means "I am"; say the *So* on the inhalation and *Ham* on the exhalation. Gradually with practice the mind will become more calm and peaceful.

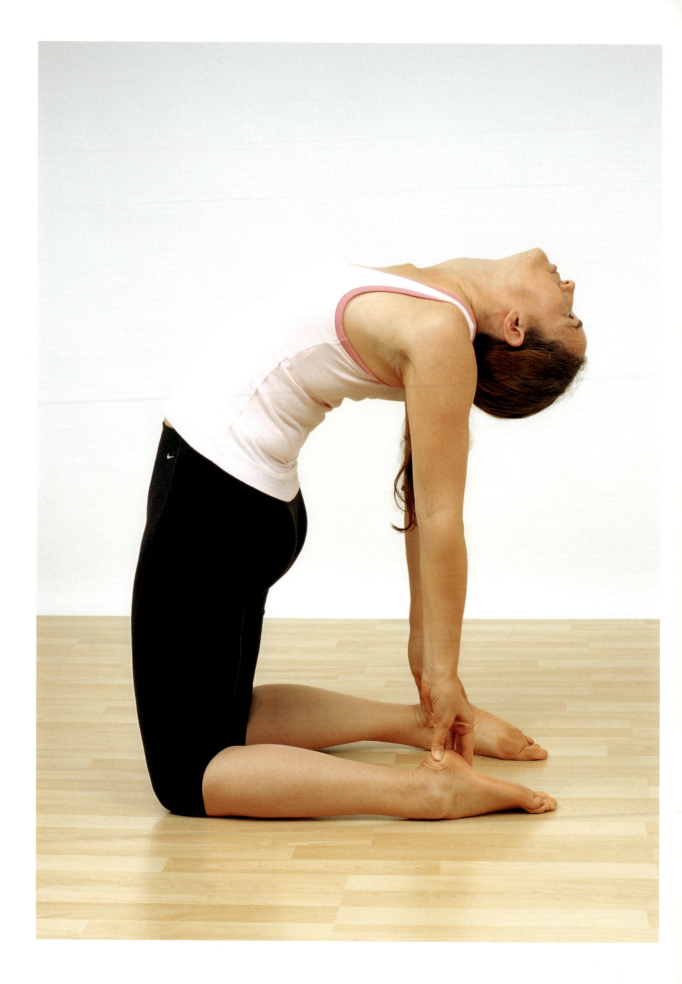

CHAPTER 5

Back-Bending

ⸯ

As we age, and after a lifetime of sitting at a desk, the back begins to round. A rounded spine constricts the lungs and affects our ability to breathe deeply. With less oxygen, the brain is starved and circulation deteriorates. Keeping the back strong and supple slows the aging process and keeps the body vital. Back-bending poses increase the space between the internal organs, removing toxins and allowing vital nutrients and blood to flow freely. Helpful for strengthening the muscles in the back, back-bends also flex the spine and stimulate the body's central energy channel. The following poses expand the chest and open the heart center, giving energy, courage, and mental clarity, which can help overcome depression.

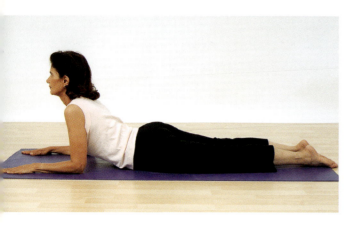

Crocodile pose *Makarasana*

Lie flat on the stomach with the feet hip-width apart. Relax the pelvis and tuck the tailbone under to lengthen the lower back. Place the hands underneath the shoulders, with the fingertips pointing forward. Place the forehead on the mat. Inhale, lift the chest and slide the forearms forward until the elbows rest directly underneath the armpits. Look straight ahead. Hold the pose for 8 breaths.

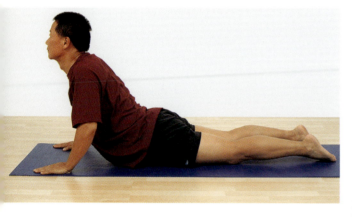

Cobra pose *Bhujangasana*

Lie flat on the stomach. Bring the feet and legs together and place the palms under the shoulders beside the rib cage. Place the forehead and then the chin on the floor. Feel the extension through the spine from the tailbone to the crown of the head. Elongate the spine, raise the head and chest and inhale. Roll the shoulders down and open the chest. Press gently into the palms, lengthening the spine vertebra by vertebra, bringing the chest forward. Keep the elbows alongside the body. Look up, without crunching in the back of the neck, and exhale. Hold for 8 breaths, breathing evenly, then exhale and release.

Half-locust pose *Ardha Salabhasana*

1. Lie face down on the mat, flat on the stomach, and place the chin on the floor. Tuck the arms under the body—have the palms either facing up or down, or make loose fists, and let them rest under the tops of the thighs.

2. Move the elbows as close together as possible. Inhale and stretch the left leg back and up. Hold for 8 breaths. Repeat on the opposite side.

> ✳ **TIP** Lift the leg as far as feels comfortable, while keeping the hip in contact with the forearm—do not force it. As you practice you will gradually be able to lift your leg higher.

1.

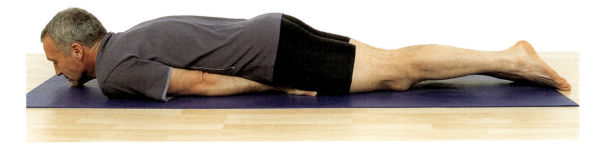

2.

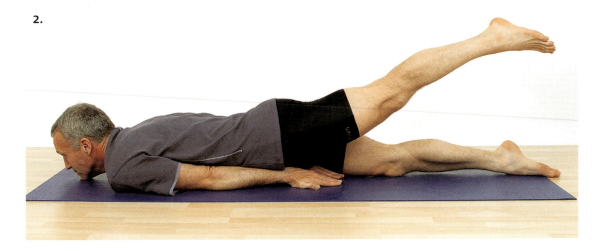

Locust pose *Salabhasana*

1. Lie flat on the stomach on the mat. Place the chin on the floor and bring the feet together. Tuck the arms under the body and shift the body weight forward into the chest and shoulders.

2. Keeping the feet and legs together, inhale, and lift both legs. Do not strain in the lower back. Hold for 8 breaths, then exhale and release the pose.

BENEFITS *Ardha salabhasana* and *salabhasana* help to keep the back strong by strengthening the muscles of the lower back, pelvis, and abdomen. They also remove tension from the wrists and elbows, and can help alleviate the symptoms of carpal tunnel syndrome. Practicing these poses will help tone the intestines and relieve constipation.

1.

2.

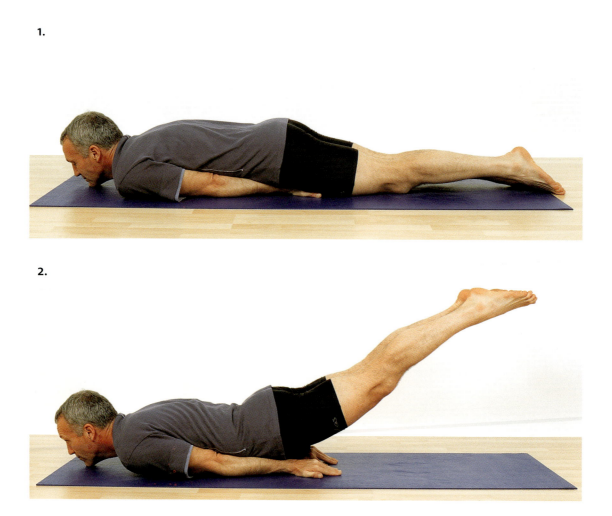

Camel pose *Ustrasana*

1. Kneel with the thighs and buttocks lifted, bringing the knees hip–width apart. Come up onto the toes. Place the hands on the lower back with fingertips pointing down, extending the spine up. Begin to lift the chest and ease the pelvis forward. Exhale as you begin to arch back.

2. Reach back one hand at a time and take hold of the heels. Keep lifting the chest.

Hold both heels and look up, without crunching in the back of the neck. Press down with the knees; keep the pelvis forward in line with the knees and the chest lifted to remove pressure from the lower back.

3. Move the shoulder blades down and into the upper back to open the chest. Extend evenly along the spine. Breathe steadily for 8 breaths. Release, holding the lower back and lifting up slowly.

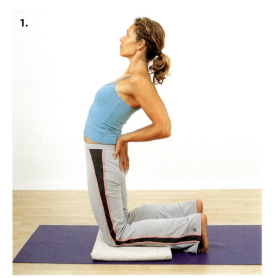

1.

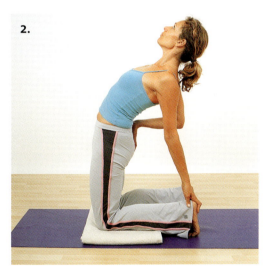

2.

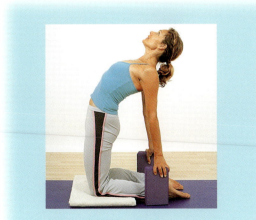

✳ **TIP** Place blocks on the outsides of the ankles. When you reach back, place the hands on the blocks for support.

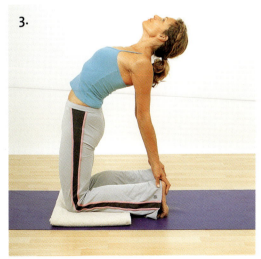

3.

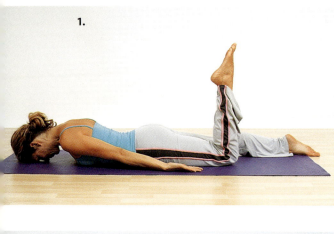

Half-bow pose *Ardha Dhanurasana*

1. Lie on your stomach, forehead on the floor and feet hip-width apart. Bend the left knee, taking the heel toward the left buttock.

2. Stretch the left arm back and take hold of the top of the left foot. Extend the right arm forward along the floor, palm down. Inhale and lift the left leg up and back. Exhale and hold for 8 breaths, breathing evenly, then repeat on the opposite side.

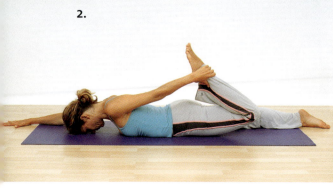

BENEFITS

Ardha dhanurasana flexes the entire spine, sending fresh blood and nutrients to the discs. The weight on the pelvis and abdomen tones the digestive and reproductive organs. *Dhanurasana* opens the chest, expands the lungs, and removes stiffness in the shoulders.

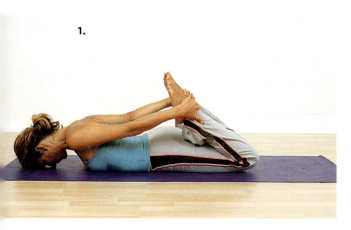

Bow pose *Dhanurasana*

1. Lie flat on the stomach. Place the forehead on the floor. Have the feet hip-width apart, bend the knees, and take the heels toward the buttocks. Stretch the arms back and take hold of the outside of the ankles. Tuck the tailbone under and place the chin on the floor. Inhale and raise the legs up and back.

2. Keep pulling up with the legs. Allow the force of the legs to lift the head and chest up as high as possible to arch the back. The spine remains passive in this pose and the shoulders relaxed.

3. Keep the arms straight as you balance on the abdomen. Raise the chin and look up without crunching the back of the neck. Exhale and breathe evenly for 8 breaths, then exhale and release the pose.

2.
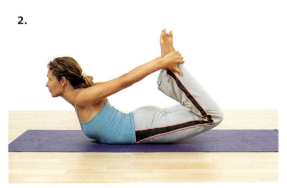

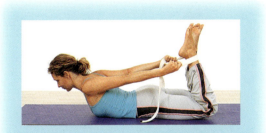

✳ **TIP** If you find it hard to reach the feet, use a belt. Place it around the ankles and hold as close to the ankles as possible, pulling the belt to lift the legs and come into the pose.

3.

Bridge pose *Setu Bandhasana*

Lie flat on your back. Bend the legs and place the soles of the feet on the floor close to the buttocks. Stretch the arms toward the feet with palms down alongside the hips. Tuck the tailbone under. Inhale. Exhale, pushing into the palms and heels, and lift the pelvis. Roll onto the tops of the shoulders if possible and lift the chest. Tuck the chin in extending through the back of the neck. Keep the thighs strong. If comfortable, reach back with the hands and interlock the fingers. Try to keep the feet parallel—if the feet turn out, it indicates stiffness in the hips. Hold for 8 breaths. Exhale and release the pose gently, placing one vertebra at a time down onto the floor.

BENEFITS *Setu bandhasana* is a useful pose for preparing for both *chakrasana* and *sarvangasana*. It opens the shoulders and the hip joints and develops flexibility in the spine. *Setu bandhasana* is especially useful for women as it helps to regulate the menstrual cycle.

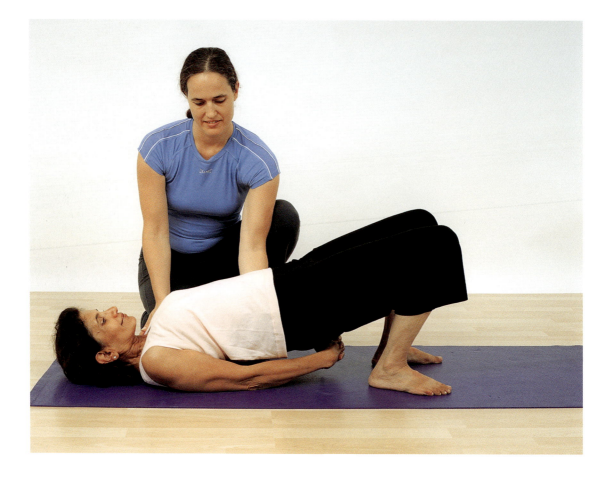

Wheel pose *Ardha Chakrasana*

1. Lie on your back. Bend the legs and place the soles of the feet on the floor close to the buttocks. Bend the elbows and place the palms of the hands flat down on the floor, underneath the shoulders. Inhale.

2. On an exhalation push into the hands and feet, raise the pelvis, and place the crown of the head on the floor. Inhale, then exhale, pushing into the palms, lifting the navel and raising the hips as high as possible. Tuck the tailbone under. Extend the chest toward the hands. Straighten the arms and keep lifting the thighs. Look down toward the floor. Breathe evenly 8 or more times, then exhale and release the pose.

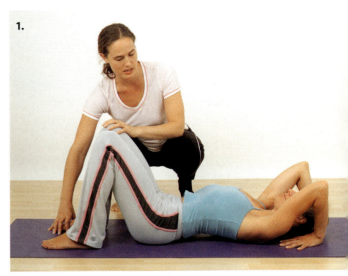

1.

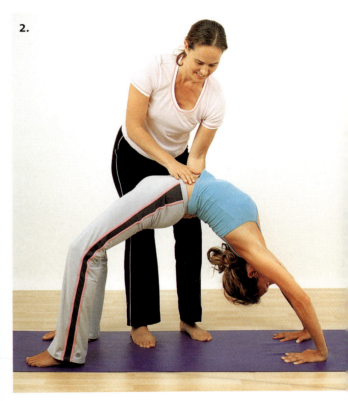

2.

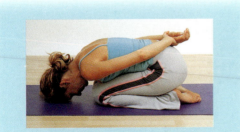

✳ **TIP** It is important after back-bending to release the spine gently in the opposite direction by coming into child's pose or gentle *paschimottanasana*.

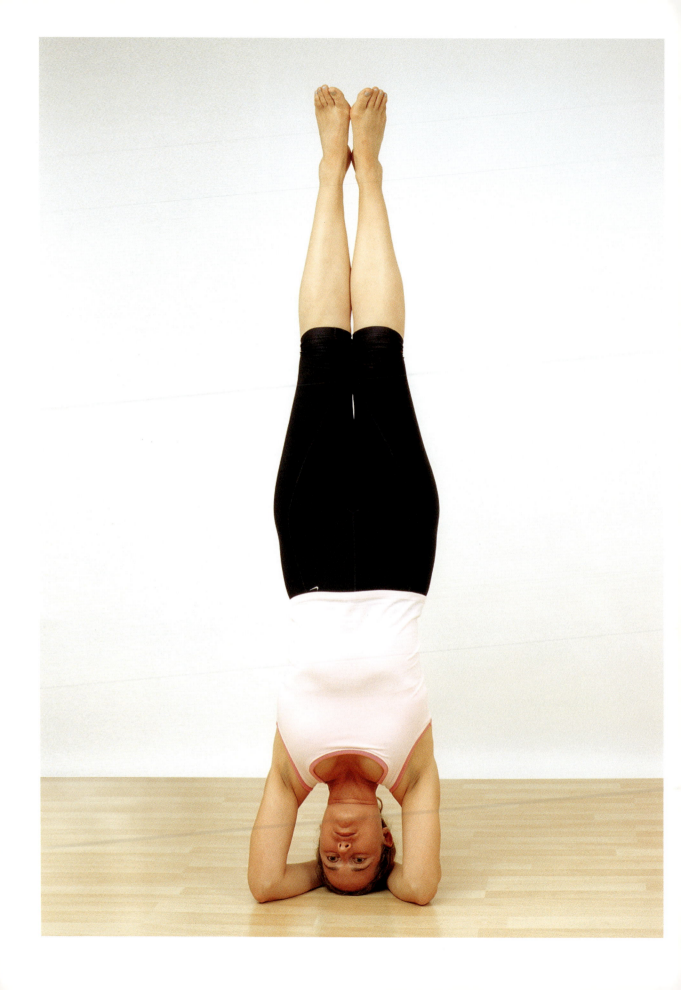

CHAPTER 6

Inversion Poses

The force of gravity asserts a constant downward pull on the body and contributes to aging. The inversions offer a welcome break and reverses the gravitational orientation of the body. Inversions send a rich supply of blood to the head and brain, which reduces wrinkles, and keeps a healthy supply of blood flowing to the brain. Turning the world upside down can help us gain a new perspective on later life. The headstand and shoulder stand are called the "king and queen of asana." because of the tremendous effect they have on the body and mind. They regulate the endocrine system, especially the pineal, pituitary, thyroid, and parathyroid glands in the head and neck, which harmonize the emotional and metabolic processes of the body by secreting hormones into the bloodstream. These inverted asanas reduce stress, anxiety, channel nervous energy, and even affect our thought processes.

Downward dog

Adho Mukha Svanasana

Lie down on the floor on your stomach. Place the palms of the hands down on the floor just below the shoulders, in line with the rib cage with the fingers pointing forward.

Make sure that the feet are hip-width apart, and tuck the toes under. Push up on to your knees. Inhale and, on an exhalation, push into the palms and raise the buttocks up and back, flattening the back of the body to form a triangle shape.

Keep the hips high and stretch the heels down to the floor, opening the backs of the knees. Look back toward the feet. Hold the pose for 8 breaths, breathing evenly, then exhale and release the pose.

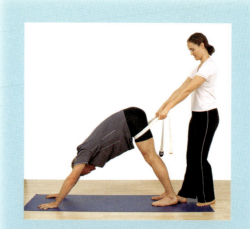

✳ **TIP** Lift the leg as far as feels comfortable, while keeping the hip in contact with the forearm—do not force it. As you practice you will gradually be able to lift your leg higher.

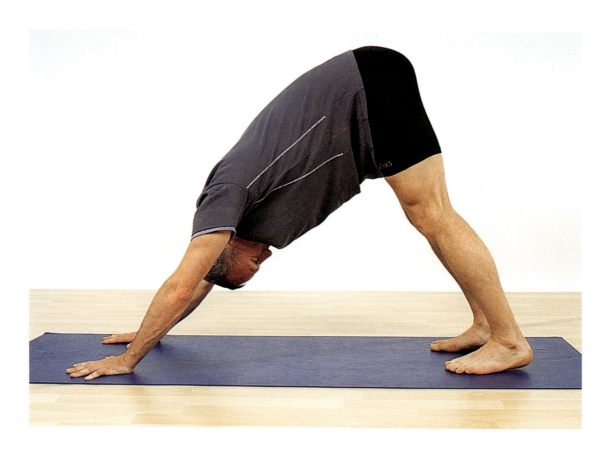

Shoulder stand with a wall

Sarvangasana

1. Lay a folded blanket close to the wall. Come into legs up the wall pose (see page 42) so the shoulder blades are flat on the blanket. Tuck the chin in, extending through the back of the neck.

2. Bend both knees and place the soles of the feet on the wall. Place arms alongside the body with the palms down, alongside the hips. Inhale.

3. Exhale, pushing against the wall with the feet and lifting the pelvis. Supporting the lower back with the hands, roll up onto the shoulder tops. Move the elbows closer for greater support.

4. Lift the feet away from the wall one foot at a time. Hold the pose for 20 to 30 seconds. To come down, bend the knees and place the feet on the wall. Exhale as you roll down one vertebra at a time.

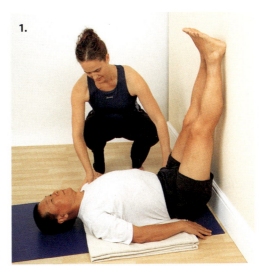

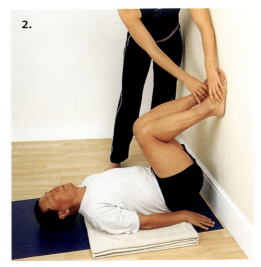

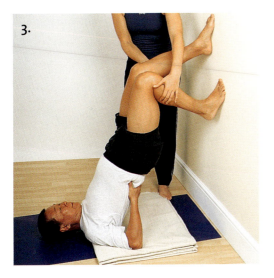

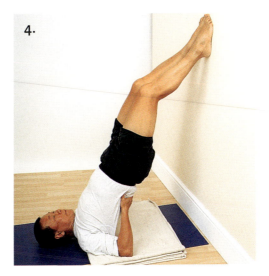

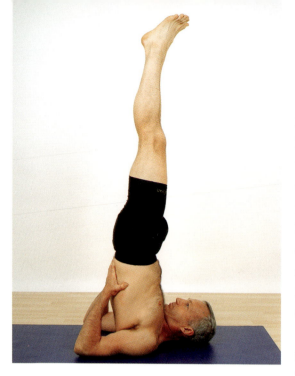

Shoulder stand *Sarvangasana*

Lie on your back. Tuck the chin in slightly and lengthen through the back of the neck. Place the arms alongside the body, with the palms down. Exhale and bend the knees, push into the palms and begin to raise the legs over the head. Bend the arms and place the hands in the middle of the back on either side of the spine to support the back without widening the elbows. Bring the torso to a vertical position, moving the chest toward the chin.

Straighten the legs to a vertical position, in line with the torso—aim for a straight line between the shoulders, hips, and ankles. Tuck the tailbone under and lengthen along the spine. Relax the muscles in the face. Inhale and breathe evenly for at least one minute. Come down or move in to *halasana*, or plow pose (see below).

BENEFITS *Sarvangasana* is the "queen" of asana: it activates the thyroid and parathyroid glands, benefiting circulation, digestion, the reproductive system, and respiration.

> ✳ **TIP** To come out of the shoulder stand and *halasana*, the plow, bend the knees toward the head, release the arms, and place them on the floor behind the body. Roll out of the pose, one vertebra at a time. Do not raise the head while coming out. Finally, release the legs to the floor and relax.

Plow pose *Halasana*

From *sarvangasana*, the shoulder stand, keep both legs together and exhale as you slowly lower them to the floor using strong abdominal muscles. Place the tips of the toes on the floor behind the head. The hips should be in line with the shoulders, and the backs of the thighs lifting toward the ceiling. Release the hands from the back, interlace the fingers, and stretch the arms away from the feet. Breathe evenly 8 or more times. Slowly roll out of the pose, or move on to the next variation.

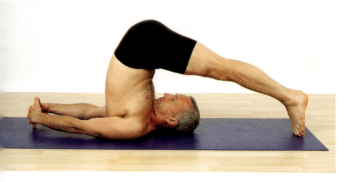

Fish pose *Matsyasana*

The fish pose should be performed after the shoulder stand as it gives a reverse stretch to the neck.

Lie on your back. Bring the legs together and tuck the hands underneath the buttocks. Push into the elbows, lift the torso, and sit up slightly to look at the feet. Lift the chest, tilt the pelvis forward, arch back, and exhale as you place the crown of the head on the floor. Relax the shoulders toward the floor. Look toward the third eye center (between the brows). Hold for 8 breaths, breathing evenly. Slowly lift out of the pose.

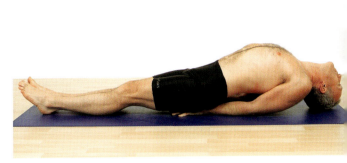

Baby headstand *Pranamasana*

1. Kneel and take hold of both heels. Tuck the chin in toward the chest and begin to curl inward, looking toward the navel. Inhale.

2. Exhale and roll forward, placing the crown of the head on the floor as close to the knees as is possible.

3. Pull on the heels and lift the hips up as high as you can; do not place too much weight on the crown. Hold for 8 breaths, breathing evenly. Exhale as you release.

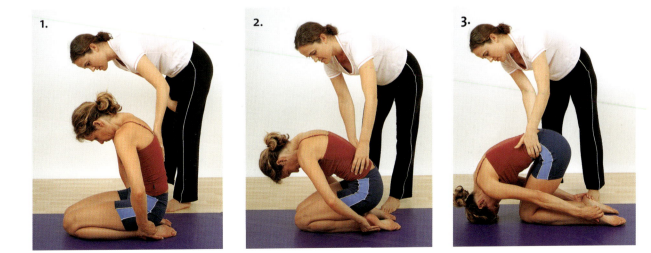

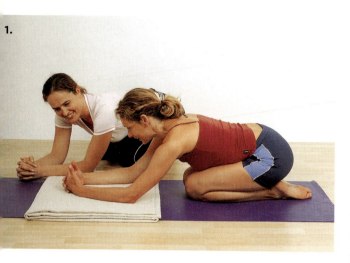

1.

Headstand *Sirsasana*

1. From a kneeling position, place the elbows on the floor underneath the shoulders. Interlace the fingers and place the heel of the hands into the floor, with the thumb pointing up, so that the arms form an equilateral triangle. Place the crown of the head down on the floor between the hands. Straighten the legs. Breathe evenly.

2. Walk the feet forward and raise the hips in line with the head. Press the forearms down and begin to distribute the weight of the body between the arms and head. Breathe.

3. Bend the knees toward the chest and raise the feet off the floor one foot at a time. As shown, if you are not confident it can help to have a partner to assist you at this stage.

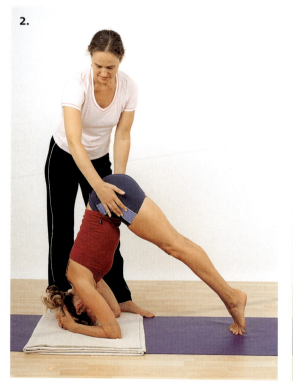

2.

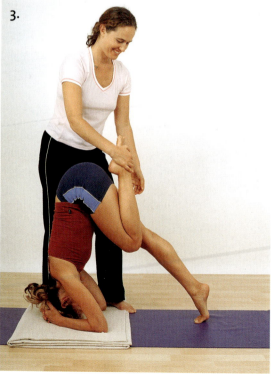

3.

4. Inhale then exhale as you slowly extend the legs. Keep pressing into the forearms, gently lift the shoulders, and tuck the tailbone under.

5. The weight of the body should be symmetrically balanced. Relax the face and allow gravity to do the work. Breathe 8 or more times, then come down slowly.

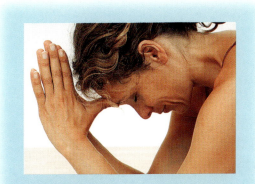

☀ **TIP** It is vital not to jump up after an inversion as the blood rushes from the head, causing dizziness. Rest in child's pose (see page 106) between inversions, or with the hands in prayer position as shown above.

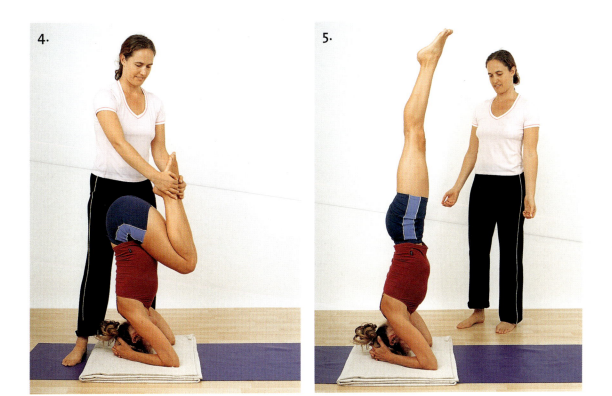

4.

5.

Relaxation Poses

Relaxation is an integral part of yoga practice. Certain poses are considered relaxation poses and can be practiced before, after, or during a yoga *asana* session. Before practicing yoga, relaxing in either *savasana* (relaxation on the back) or *shankhasana* (child's pose) allows the body to release the stresses and strains of the day and to soothe the nervous system, preparing it for the session ahead. The same two yoga poses, along with *advasana* (relaxation on the belly) can be practiced at any point during a session if you become tired. At the end of practice it is essential to spend 10 to 15 minutes lying in *savasana,* for deep relaxation. Deep relaxation, termed *yoga nidra* or "yoga sleep," allows the benefits of the yoga *asana* session to be assimilated. *Yoga nidra* is a very difficult practice, as it is not a matter of just spacing out but rather a very conscious physical letting go while the mind remains clear and alert.

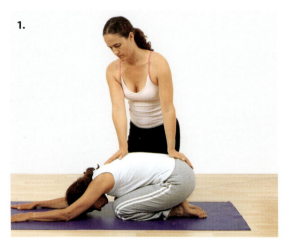

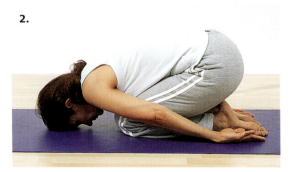

Child's pose *Shankhasana*

Child's pose can be practiced at any time, although it is particularly useful to do after back-bending to relieve tension in the lower back, or after inversions to allow time for the body to center.

1. Kneel on the mat. Slowly fold forward and place the forehead on the floor. Try to maintain the contact between the buttocks and the heels.

2. Take the arms back so that the hands are alongside the body, in line with the heels, with the backs of the hands resting on the floor. If the head does not touch the floor then place the forehead on a block. Breathe and relax the belly. Feel the abdomen pressing against the thighs on the inhale, and releasing on the exhale. Rest for a few minutes.

Relaxation on the belly *Advasana*

Resting on the belly is particularly useful between prone back-bending poses like dhanurasana *(the bow) or* salabhasana *(the locust).*

Lie on your stomach and turn the head to one side. Place the arms alongside the body, with the backs of the hands touching the floor and the palms upward. Breathe steadily, and let the belly relax. Feel the abdomen pressing against the floor on the inhalation, and releasing on the exhalation. Rest for a few minutes.

Relaxation on the back *Savasana*

During savasana *it is important not to move the body at all, as even the slightest movement creates muscular tension.*

Lie flat on the back, with the head and spine in a straight line. Move the feet about hip-distance apart and allow the feet to drop to the sides. Place the arms a few inches from the body with the palms facing up and the fingers relaxed. Tuck the chin in slightly and relax the face. Close the eyes, and allow the corners of the eyes to release and let go. Scan the body for any tension. If you observe any tension then squeeze that part of the body tightly for few moments and let go. Once the body is relaxed make a commitment not to move. Become aware of the natural breath and allow it to become rhythmic and relaxed. If the mind wanders and becomes busy then gently bring it back to the breath. Rest for 10 minutes. To come out of relaxation, begin to deepen the breath, very gently move the fingers and toes. Take a long deep stretch. Bend the knees into the chest, and roll to the right side in a fetal position. Slowly come up to stand.

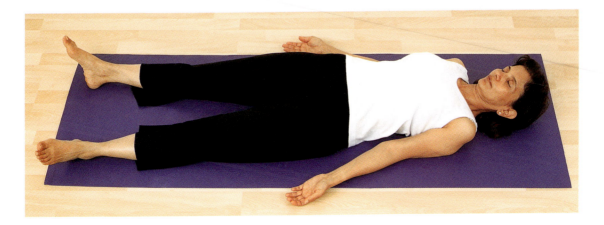

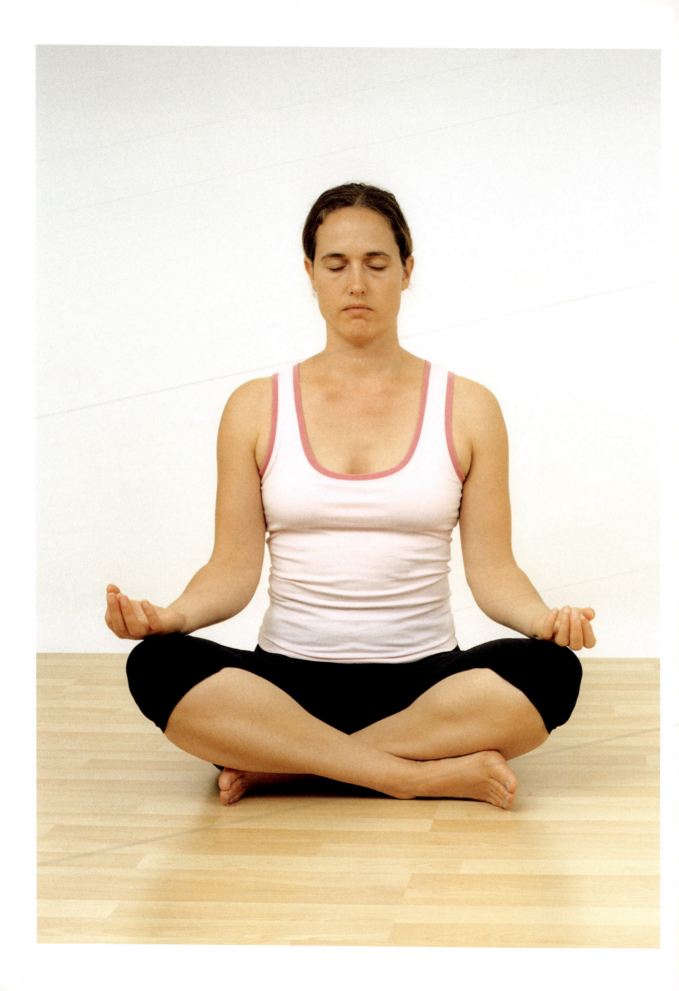

CHAPTER 7

Asanas for Ailments

Symptoms of aging, from increased body fat, stiffness in the joints and high blood pressure to brittle bones and heart disease, are not inevitable. Research indicates that age-related problems can be due to poor diet, lack of exercise, and high levels of stress. By improving your diet and taking a common-sense approach to maintaining fitness through yoga, you can become stronger, increase flexibility, have more energy, and develop a positive outlook. Yoga is unique in that the movements and techniques can be adjusted to suit each person's situation and ability. For example, during menopause the need for physically demanding yoga practice is replaced here with restorative poses to help balance the change of life. Yoga practice teaches us to "be," to become increasingly sensitive to the body and mind and release preconceived notions and expectations.

Eyes

TO RELIEVE EYESTRAIN AND IMPROVE VISION

Age can bring changes that may weaken your eyes, making reading in particular more difficult. The eyes are designed to see a range of distances, both near and far. However, many occupations involve fixing the eyes on one plane for extended periods of time, like looking at a computer screen. The eyes are a part of the nervous system, so when the eyes become tired it creates internal stress.

Yoga recognizes the importance of caring for the eyes to maintain accurate vision and to relax the nervous system. Eye professionals agree that adequate rest and relaxation are very important for the proper care of your eyes. Stress and strain result in a build-up of pressure on the optic nerve, the eye muscles, and the retina as well as causing changes in the flow of blood in the veins that supply blood to the eyes.

Bathing the eyes in warm sunlight, by sitting with your face toward the sun with the eyes closed for 10 minutes, helps to release tension. The warmth of the sunlight will increase the flow of blood in your eyes and stimulate the nerve cells in your eyes. Diet is also important, eating plenty of vegetables and food items that contain Vitamin A, like eggs, milk, leafy vegetables, and carrots.

Yoga exercises for the eyes help to strengthen the eye muscles, tone the optic nerves, and relieve eyestrain. If practiced regularly these three exercises have been found to improve eyesight.

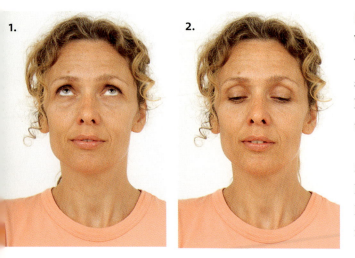

1.

2.

Eye exercises *Netra Vyaayaamam*
VERTICAL MOVEMENTS

1. Sit in a comfortable seated position either on a chair or on the floor. Center the eyes. Inhale, look up toward the eyebrows, without moving the head.

2. Exhale and drop the eyes to look down. Keep the vision soft and the movements fluid. Repeat 10 to 20 times. Close the eyes and rest for a few moments.

HORIZONTAL MOVEMENTS

1. Sit in a comfortable seated position either on a chair or on the floor. Center the eyes. Exhale and sweep the eyes all the way to the your right.

2. Inhale and move the eyes in a straight horizontal line to your left. Repeat 10 to 20 times. Close the eyes and rest.

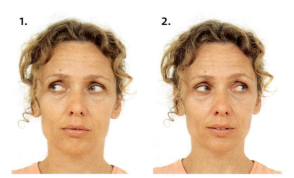

CIRCULAR MOVEMENTS

Sit in a comfortable position. Center the eyes. Imagine that there is a large clock face in front of you. Start by looking up toward twelve o'clock and move your eyes counterclockwise counting down every number on the clock from twelve to eleven and so on all the way around. Move the eyes slowly and smoothly like the second hand of a clock, touching every point around the periphery of the eyes. Repeat 4 to 10 times in both directions.

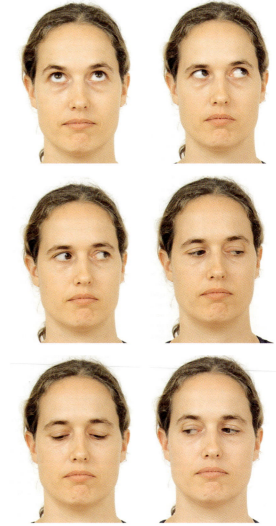

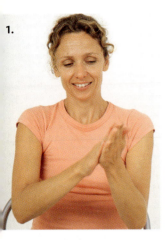

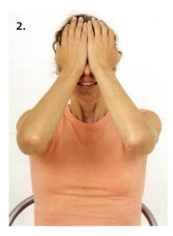

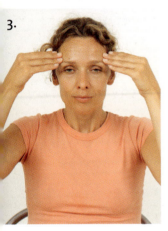

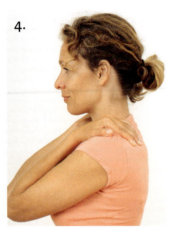

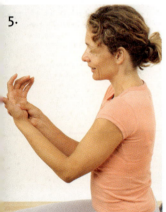

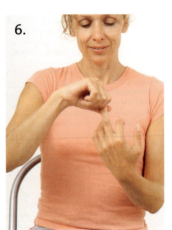

Post–eye exercise massage

1. Bring the hands into prayer position. Rub the palms together briskly until they feel hot.

2. Cup the palms over the eyes and bathe the eyes in the heat and darkness.

3. Massage the forehead and brow with the fingertips to release any tension around the eyes.

4. Then take the hands to the back of the neck and gently squeeze any tension from the neck and shoulders. Take hold of the opposite shoulder with each hand and continue massaging down the arms.

5. Gently squeeze and massage each palm with a circular thumb motion.

6. Softly pull the tip of each finger, to release tension through the hands and to loosen the joints.

Feet

ༀ

The feet are often the most neglected and misused part of our anatomy. After decades of stuffing them into tight, ridiculously shaped shoes, it is no wonder that in later life the feet finally break down. Over the age of 40, as many as 80 percent of people have some type of foot problem, with women having four times as many problems as men.

The feet are an architectural wonder. The twenty-six bones in the feet are able to support and cushion the entire body weight, and to propel the body through space. The condition of the feet impacts the entire structure and alignment of the body. For instance, when we wear high-heeled shoes, the entire body weight is thrown forward onto the ball of the foot, causing the back to bend backward in order to compensate, resulting in numerous structural misalignments causing hip, knee, or back problems. Also the ankle is not properly supported and becomes weak and more prone to sprains and falls.

The beauty of yoga is that it is practiced in bare feet, giving a greater connection with the earth, which helps us to feel grounded. Numerous nerve endings in the feet correspond to each gland, organ, and part of the body, so massaging the feet relaxes and normalizes all the body's functions, restoring natural balance. Also, there are more sweat glands on the feet than anywhere else, so allowing air to circulate and the feet to breathe is a good practice.

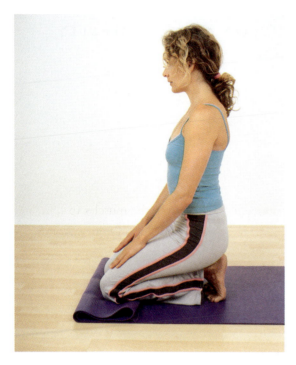

Foot exercises

The following yoga exercises help to stretch the feet and maintain flexibility in the toes.

Sitting toe strengthener

Come into a kneeling position. Stand up on both knees, with the knees hip-width apart and the toes tucked under. Sit back and place the buttocks on top of the heels. Hold for 20 seconds and release.

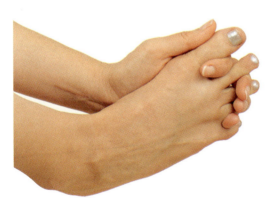

Toe stretching

Sit comfortably on a chair or the floor. Bend the right leg and place the right ankle on top of the left thigh, close to the left knee. Relax the right knee out to the side. Carefully insert the fingers between each toe, to create space between the toes. Hold for a few minutes. Repeat with the opposite foot.

Easing the Symptoms of Arthritis

Contrary to old beliefs, it is now recognized that arthritis sufferers need to remain active. When we are inactive, the muscles atrophy and it becomes increasingly harder to move, which triggers a negative downward spiral of inactivity, depression, and lethargy.

YOGA BENEFITS

Yoga has been shown to reduce the symptoms of arthritis, and is being used more and more for pain management. The movements help to increase joint mobility and to strengthen the muscles that support the body, which increases joint stability. Without exercise, the bones become brittle, leaving sufferers at greater risk of injury due to a fall. The yoga asanas strengthen the bones and restore agility and poise. The breathing and meditation practices also help to calm the nervous system, which helps people to cope with pain more effectively.

However, when beginning an exercise program it is important to respect pain. A stretching pain is good, but if sharp pain is experienced, always stop the exercise and rest. Never bounce in a pose as it can damage ligaments and tear muscles. Try to make the movements as fluid as possible following the natural line of motion of the joint. As an arthritis sufferer your range of motion may be limited, but in order to maintain joint mobility it is important to move each joint within its comfortable range.

Breathe steadily and evenly to send as much oxygen to the joints as possible, as this helps them perform at their best. Never hold your breath; we tend to hold the breath when concentrating, causing the muscles to tense and shorten, which may result in injury. Working in a heated room or having a hot bath or shower before practicing helps prepare the muscles and joints for the movements.

HOW TO PRACTICE

The following 35-minute program includes simple warm-up exercises that are gentle and restorative for arthritis sufferers. The exercises should be practiced regularly when pain and stiffness are at a minimum. For rheumatoid arthritis sufferers who tend to be stiff in the morning, an afternoon session is advisable: for osteoarthrhitis sufferers, who tend to get stiffer as the day progresses, a morning session is better. Getting started, especially when experiencing pain, is one of the most difficult hurdles. Begin slowly and rest between poses if necessary.

CAUTION

Yoga is not a substitute for allopathic or other medical therapies; rather, it is a complementary treatment to help alleviate the symptoms of disease. It is advisable to show this routine to your physician or physical therapist to determine the type and amount of exercise that it right for you.

Asanas to help arthritis

Many of the following exercises can be practiced sitting on a firm chair.

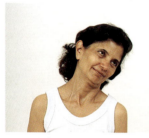

Head rolls (see p 49)

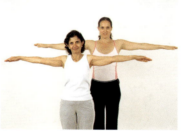

Shoulder circles (see p 50)

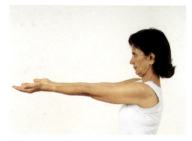

Elbow bends (see p 51)

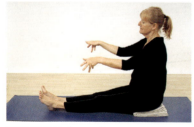

Wrist rotations (see p 51)

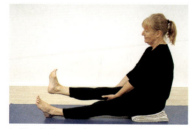

Ankle rolls (see p 51)

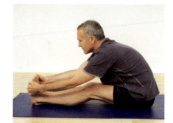

Forward bend (see p 81)

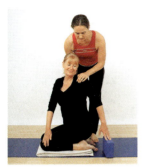

Side twist (see p 86)

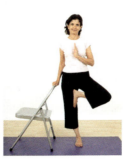

Eagle pose (see p 53)

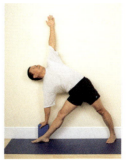

Tree pose with a chair (see p 32)

Triangle pose with block (see p 34)

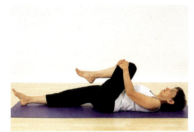

One knee to chest (see p 76)

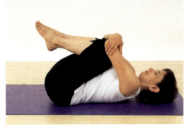

Both knees to chest (see p 76)

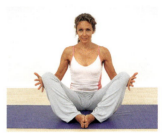

Cobbler pose (see p 84)

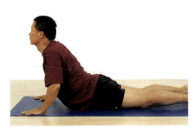

Cobra pose (see p 90)

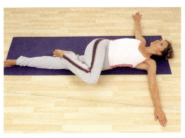

Lying side stretch (see p 78)

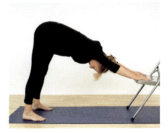

Downward dog with a chair (see p 32)

Getting Up and Down to the Floor

After a lifetime of sitting in chairs it becomes increasingly difficult to get down to the floor, which is necessary for many yoga postures. The action of getting up and down from the floor helps to keep the joints healthy and the body limber. For practitioners that are new to yoga or are suffering with arthritis, it is important to move slowly and safely to avoid injury.

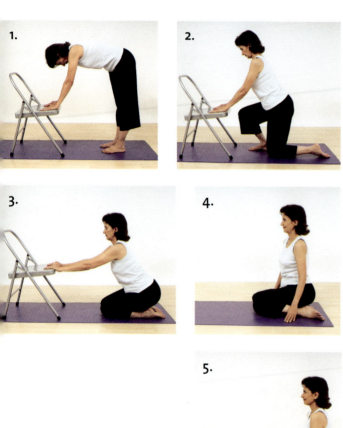

Getting down to the floor with a chair

1. Place a chair on the yoga mat, to prevent it from slipping, with the seat facing you. Stand in front of the chair about 2 feet (0.6 m) away. Bend forward and place your hands on the front of the chair.

2. Step the right foot forward. Supporting your body weight with your arms, slowly bend the left knee down on to the floor.

3. Bend the right knee in line with the left and come to a kneeling position. Release the chair.

4. Lift the hips and take them to one side of the feet. Placing the hands down on the floor for additional support.

5. Swing the legs to one side, away from the hips. Extend the legs out in front with the feet together. To get up from the floor with the support of a chair, repeat the movements in the opposite direction.

Getting up from lying position

Lying flat on your back in *Savasana* is the final pose at the end of a yoga session.

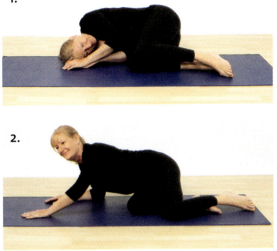

1. Bend the knees into the chest and roll to the right side. Rest for a few moments in a fetal position.

2. Place the left hand down onto the mat in front of the chest. Press into the left hand and begin to lift the torso up.

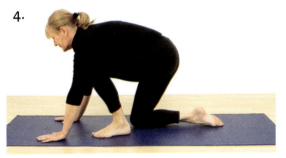

3. Come up onto your hands and knees and find your balance.

4. Bend the left knee and place the sole of the foot on the floor close to the hands.

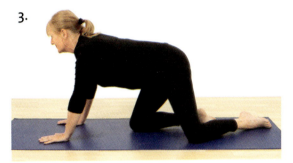

5. Begin to shift the body weight into the hands and left foot and until you can step the right foot forward in line with the left. From a crouched position shift the body weight into both feet. Slowly come up to a standing position.

6. Stand in *tadasana* for a few moments to find your center.

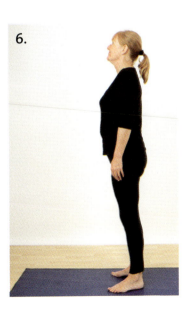

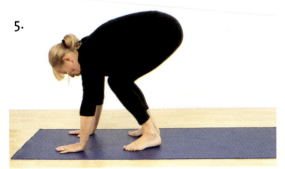

Helping the Symptoms of Heart Disease

❧

Yoga is an amazing technique not only for working on the physical body but also on the deeper internal energy body. In the U.S. in 1990, a doctor named Dean Ornish first published his groundbreaking study showing that making lifestyle changes, including a healthy yoga diet, yoga exercise, meditation and positive thinking, can help heart disease. For one year, he treated a group of patients suffering with chronic heart disease with a program that included an hour a day of yoga, deep relaxation, meditation, and a vegetarian diet. By practicing yoga daily, his patients were able to reverse heart disease without the use of drugs and avoid bypass surgery.

WHAT ARE THE CONTRIBUTORY FACTORS

As we age various changes take place in the body, which may contribute to heart disease. Cholesterol, especially bad cholesterol (low-density lipoprotein, or LDL) increases; too much can cause clogged arteries and high blood pressure, which is another contributory factor in heart disease. Being overweight also puts us at higher risk, because the body has to work much harder to pump blood around the body.

However, the good news is that exercise reduces the level of bad cholesterol in the system and increases the good cholesterol. A healthy diet rich in vegetables, fruits, and grains is essential to prevent heart disease. Eating fewer saturated fats also helps prevent excessive weight gain.

HEALING STRESS

Stress is also a major contributor to heart disease. Deep relaxation during yoga induces a state of homeostasis, or balance, in the body, which helps to reduce stress. During breathing exercises, the heart accelerates on inhalation and slows on exhalation, so an extended exhalation helps to slow the heart and reduce blood pressure. When we do not breathe rhythmically, the heart is put under high stress.

PURIFYING THE HEART

According to yoga philosophy, another important dimension to the heart concerns the subtle energy body, the *nadis* or energy channels that form a network across the entire body (see page 17). At the heart center, the left and right channels are entwined particularly tightly around the central channel. The energy flowing in the inner channels, especially the left and right channels, is very connected to how we think. When we have strong negative emotions, the left and right channels swell and choke the central channel and block vital energy from flowing freely, thereby starving the heart. Yoga aims to purify negative emotions and reawaken the heart to experience the world with the freedom, innocence, and openness of a young child.

Asanas to help heart disease

The following *asanas* may help to relieve the symptoms of heart disease.

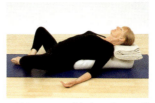
Cobbler pose with bolster (see p 28)

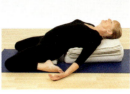
Hero pose with bolster (see p 29)

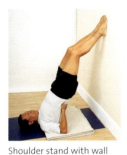
Shoulder stand with wall (see p 101)

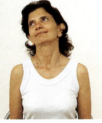
Head rolls (see p 49)

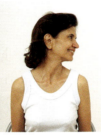
Head turns (see p 48)

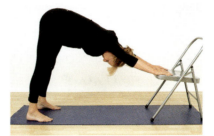
Downward dog with a chair (see p 32)

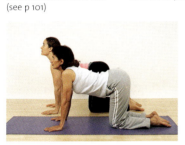
Cat pose (see p 52)

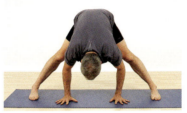
Extended leg pose (see p 68)

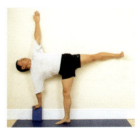
Half-moon pose (see p 43)

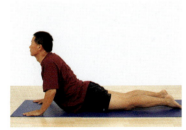
Cobra pose (see p 90)

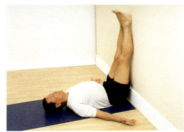
Legs up the wall (see p 42)

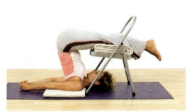
Plow pose with a chair (see p 33)

✳ **CAUTION** When suffering from heart disease it is important not to raise the arms over shoulder height.

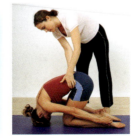
Baby head stand (see p 103)

To Restore the Body's Balance During Menopause

❦

Menopause is part of the natural life cycle, which ushers in a new phase in a woman's existence. The change of life, when menstruation stops, is caused by a shift in hormone production. Perimenopause, or fluctuation in hormone production, starts a few years before menopause, between 45 and 55. This hormone flux can produce symptoms such as hot flashes, night sweats, insomnia, irritability, depression, and mood swings. These uncomfortable side-effects have created a general misconception of menopause as an age-related disease, which has prompted the medical community to produce a range of medications to help ease these effects.

HORMONE REPLACEMENT THERAPY

The main medication given to women over 45 is HRT, or hormone replacement therapy. After menopause, the ovaries produce less estrogen and progesterone, which the body requires to keep bones healthy and the body vital. Scientists believed that maintaining hormone levels at the old rate with a replacement hormone from mare's urine would remove the symptoms of menopause and actually slow the aging process. However, recent research has revealed that HRT may not be the miracle answer to eternal youth. HRT has been shown to increase the risk of cancer, particularly breast and endometrial cancer, and can cause blood clots. Increasing the level of progesterone, the sister hormone to estrogen, which helps to reduce the risk of cancer, has been found to increase the risk of heart disease, stroke, and cardiovascular problems.

MENOPAUSE AND LIFESTYLE

Each woman experiences menopause differently, and it is interesting to note that in other cultures where lifestyle follows a more natural rhythm, menopausal symptoms are practically nonexistent. Due to the many side-effects of replacement hormones, doctors now encourage women to pursue a healthy lifestyle, including a diet rich in fruit and vegetables, and exercises to strengthen the bones and heart. A number of natural plant supplements have been shown to prevent the symptoms of menopause including flaxseed oil, evening primrose oil, vitamin B6, vitamin E, and vitamin C. Eating soy is particularly good as it is high in a natural plant form of estrogen.

Menstrual cycles are governed by the endocrine system, especially the pituitary gland in the brain, which triggers the ovaries to produce estrogen and progesterone. Post-menopause, when the ovaries produce less estrogen, the adrenal glands take over and produce a form of estrogen called esterone, to maintain healthy bones. The practices of yoga are designed to stimulate the endocrine glands and keep them in good working order, thus helping to make the transitions of life smooth and symptom free. The more we are able to embrace the change of life the easier the transition. Many women find post-menopause to be a time of renewed vigor, energy, and freedom.

The following yoga exercises are recommended to ease the particular discomforts associated with menopause. Yoga aims to purify negative emotions and reawaken the heart to experience the world with the freedom, innocence, and openness of a young child.

For hot flashes and night sweats

Hot flashes are one of the most common symptoms of menopause where the body temperature rises causing the face, neck, and arms to blush. Supported forward bends are particularly recommended, as they are cooling and help calm the nervous system. Reclining poses like *supta baddhakonasana* and *supta virasana* help to open the chest, which improves breathing and also releases tension in the pelvis. Avoid eating spicy food, coffee, alcohol, and hot drinks as they create heat in the body.

To help anxiety and insomnia

During menopause, because of erratic hormone production, you can feel jittery and nervous, and suffer from anxiety and insomnia. The following poses help to calm the nervous system and restore harmony.

RESTORATIVE POSES

Restorative poses are particularly recommended for menopause, to help nourish and restore balance to the body. Restorative poses are postures that are practiced with the support of various props, which include a chair or wall, blocks, blankets, a belt or bolster, and are held for a few minutes. The props support the body in a posture, allowing you to relax more deeply into the pose. It is important to feel comfortable in a pose and, as each person's body has unique proportions, you will need to experiment to find the perfect height and placement of your prop.

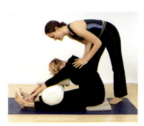
Forward bend with a bolster (see p 30)

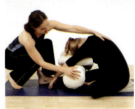
Head-to-knee pose with a bolster (see p 30)

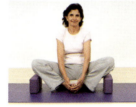
Cobbler pose with blocks (see p 35)

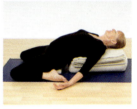
Hero pose with bolster (see p 29)

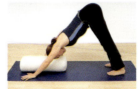
Downward dog with bolster (see p 29)

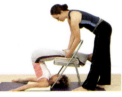
Plow pose with a chair (see p 33)

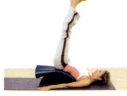
Half-shoulder stand with a back arch (see p 45)

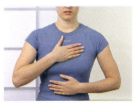
Full yogic breath (see p 22)

To relieve fatigue

The internal changes during menopause can often result in a general malaise. The following *asanas* are good for overcoming fatigue.

Legs up the wall, or *vaparita karani,* can help you feel grounded if you're suffering from a bout of indecision. It is one of the most healing of the yoga poses, reducing the heart rate and promoting deep relaxation. It is also good for mild hypertension.

Gentle, supported back-bends help to stimulate the adrenal glands and lift the spirits, try the following exercises for increased vitality.

Muddled thoughts

The mind often gets cloudy and muddled during menopause, resulting in indecisiveness. To help improve the functioning of the mind inversions are highly recommended along with deep breathing to send oxygen and nutrients to the brain, though it is not recommended to practice inversions during menstruation.

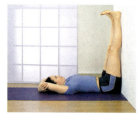

Legs up the wall (see p 42)

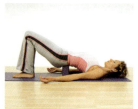

Bridge pose with a block (see p 35)

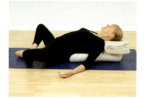

Cobbler pose with a bolster (see p 28)

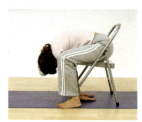

Forward bend with a chair (see p 31)

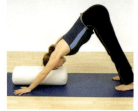

Downward dog with a bolster (see p 29)

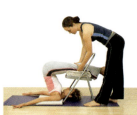

Plow pose with a chair (see p 33)

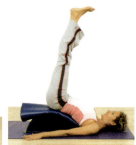

Half-shoulder stand with a back arch (see p 45) or Shoulder stand with a blanket (see p 36)

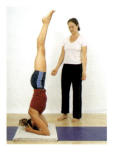

Headstand (see p 104)

> ### HERBS FOR HORMONE BALANCE
> The following herbs help balance progesterone/estrogen levels: alfalfa, Chinese ginseng, licorice root, raspberry leaves and fennel.

OSTEOPOROSIS

One of the most chronic diseases that can be a by-product of post-menopause is osteoporosis. Brittle bones, or reduced bone density due to reduced levels of progesterone and estrogen, characterizes osteoporosis. In the US, 10 million people suffer from osteoporosis, 80 percent of whom are post-menopausal women. Osteoporosis can progress painlessly until a bone breaks. The areas of the body that are most susceptible are the hip, spine, and wrists. A hip fracture almost always requires hospitalization and major surgery. Spinal fractures can result in a loss of height, severe back pain, and deformity.

However, osteoporosis in not an inevitable result of menopause. Recommended prevention for osteoporosis focuses on a healthy diet and proper exercise. A healthy balanced diet is one rich in nutrients. For people suffering from osteoporosis, the intake of calcium from dairy products, especially yogurt and cheese, is recommended, along with collard greens and broccoli. Vitamin D is another essential nutrient that increases calcium absorption. It can be best absorbed by sitting in the sun for 15 minutes a day. Fish oil is another good source of Vitamin D. Cutting out cigarettes and alcohol is also advisable as both activities increase the likelihood of brittle bones, while salt leeches calcium from the bones so is also best avoided.

Exercise, especially weight-bearing exercises, are essential in the prevention of osteoporosis. When we place weight on a particular limb, the muscles send a message to the bone causing it to thicken and become strong. Another advantage of regular exercise is that the muscles get firmer, which act as a shock absorber and can cushion a fall, preventing bone damage.

Yoga is a great weight-bearing form of exercise, as the poses redistribute the weight to various parts of the body in a safe and gentle way, allowing the body to build up more strength over time. Balancing poses and inversions are especially bone-strengthening exercises, placing the body weight on one leg, or the head or hands, for example. They also improve overall balance and agility in later life. The ability to balance is one of the last motor-neuron skills we learn as children and one of the first to go in later life, so it is important to prolong the ability through regular practice.

Stress is also a contributing factor to osteoporosis, as it creates acidity in the blood that contributes to bone depletion. The breathing techniques, meditation, and deep relaxation are useful in reducing stress and making the blood more alkaline, which is better for internal health.

GLOSSARY

Amma Accumulated toxins, undigested food, and waste material in the body.

Anandamaya Kosha The field of limitless potential.

Annamaya Kosha The physical body.

Asana Yoga posture. Literally, "steady, comfortable pose."

Chakras Energy centers. Literally, "wheels."

Dandasana Staff pose; the neutral sitting pose for all forward bends.

Kapalabhati breathing Rapid diaphragmatic breathing that removes impurities from the body.

Manomaya Kosha The mind body.

Nadis Energy channels that form a network across our entire bodies; the channels radiating energy from the chakras.

Prana Energy; life force. Referred to as *chi* by the Chinese.

Pranamaya Kosha The energy body.

Pranayama Breathing exercises that rhythmically control the breath. Literally, "expansion of the life force."

Savasana Relaxation on the back. Gives the body time to absorb the full benefits of the practice.

Surya Namaskar Sun salutation; a dynamic series of fourteen asanas linked together with the breath.

Tadasana Primary standing pose that teaches realignment and balance.

Ujjai breathing Breathing technique whereby you gently contract the glottis to produce a soft snoring sound at the back of the throat.

Vijnanamaya Kosha Awareness.

Yoga Union. To yoke or to join; to attach the mind to one object and to penetrate its essential nature.

Yoga Nidra Deep relaxation, or "yoga sleep." Allows the benefits of the asanas to be assimilated.

INDEX